Ayurvedic Yoga Therapy

Mukunda Stiles

LOTUS
PRESS

P.O. Box 325
Twin Lakes, WI 53181 USA

First Edition 2007
Reprinted 2010
Reprinted 2016
Reprinted 2020

Printed in the United States of America

ISBN   978-0-9409-8597-1

Library of Congress Catalog Number   2007933732

Cover photo of Mukunda in Virabhadrasana II (Warrior Pose) by Dean Krakel

Image of Patanjali on the chapter heading pages given to Mukunda by BKS Iyengar

LOTUS PRESS

Published by:
Lotus Press, P.O. Box 325, Twin Lakes, WI 53181 USA
web: www.lotuspress.com
Email: lotuspress@lotuspress.com
800.824.6396

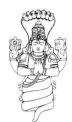

Correction: *Balancing Tree Vinyasa page 117 continued...*

Balancing Tree Vinyasa
Vrksasana
Mukunda Tom Stiles © 1991

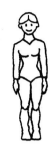 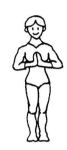 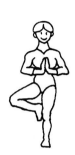 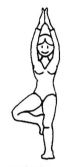 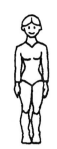

1. INHALE in Mountain Pose Tadasana

2. INHALE palms to Namaste

3. EXHALE right foot to left knee

4. INHALE arms up namaste Tree Pose - Vrksasana

5. EXHALE lower hands & leg. Reverse side, 2-5.

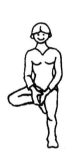 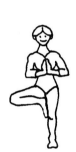 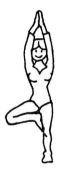 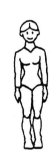

6. EXHALE right heel to groin.

7. INHALE palms to Namaste EXHALE then

8. INHALE arms up Namaste

9. EXHALE lower hands & leg. Reverse side, 6-9. INHALE then

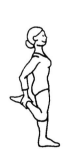 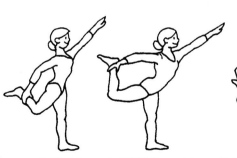 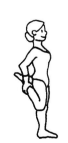

10. EXHALE right heel to hip

11. INHALE left arm up EXHALE then

12. INHALE extend chest, lift knee. EXHALE – Dancer King Natarajasana

13. INHALE, erect heel to hip.

14. EXHALE both hands pull heel to hip.

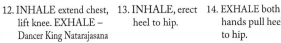

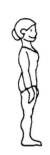 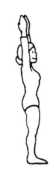 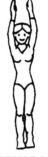 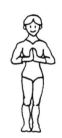

15. EXHALE release foot. Reverse side 10-14

16. INHALE arms up shoulder width apart

17. EXHALE lower hips ⅓. Squeeze thighs INHALE then

18. EXHALE half squat INHALE then

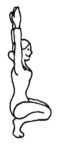 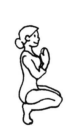 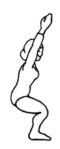 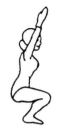

19. EXHALE full squat balance on toes.

20. INHALE namaste Squat pose - Utkatasana

21. INHALE full upright position arms overhead.

22. EXHALE namaste to your heart.

Yoga Therapy Center

BLESSINGS

These teachings draw from 36 years of teachings and reflections from Tirumalai Krishnamacharya, who while not my direct teacher, was the master of my major teachers. Paul Copeland, MD who first exposed me to his love of Narayan through Vinyasas personally given him for yoga therapy by the master in private instruction 1971-73. Through Paul's blessings I met Rama Jyoti Vernon who has remained a steadfast friend and my teacher of Classical Yoga since 1974. From her blessings I was introduced to Mataji Indra Devi (the first Lady of Yoga), BKS Iyengar, and TKV Desikachar.

Most profound gratitude to my guru Swami Muktananda Paramahansa who brought about a spiritual awakening, renamed me and gave me the seva of being a professional yogi in 1974. And to my spiritual teachers Swami Prakashananda of Suptashring and Amritanandamayi Ma (Ammachi) who keep me on this Yoga path during the extremes of difficulty and bliss.

From these great masters I have lived a life of blessings and was shown how to spread those blessings.

CONTENTS PAGE

I. Yoga and Ayurveda

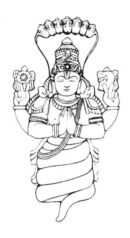

Yoga and Ayurveda belong to each other like a brother to his sister, the breath to the body, a plant in its soil. Taken in context, each one nourishes the other; removed from each other, they can exist for awhile but will lack the feeling of wholeness and continuity and will ultimately perish. Yoga has been known in the West for over one hundred years, yet it has only been in the past few decades that Ayurveda has come to be studied. Ayurveda and Yoga are sister sciences of the Indian Vedic tradition known as the Sanatana Dharma, paths to the Eternal Truth. The teachings are considered timeless as they apply to everyone in all cultures and times. By the practice of the lifestyles they recommend, life becomes more fulfilling. The goal of this book is to help you understand Ayurveda and Yoga sufficiently, leading you to specific Classical Yoga practices that have the potential to bring about a lasting change in your lifestyle, health, and overall outlook on the purpose of life.

David Frawley, a preeminent authority on Vedic culture has written that "Ayurveda is the Vedic science of healing for both body and mind. Yoga is the Vedic science of Self-realization that depends upon a well-functioning body and mind." [1] Yoga builds upon the foundation of Ayurveda and similarly Ayurveda alone is unfulfilling to the human psyche as it evolves toward Self-realization. The practice of the two sciences as a lifestyle is necessary for the achievement of their independent goals. "Yoga rests upon Ayurvedic medicine for its health implications. Ayurveda rests upon Yoga for its mental and spiritual dimension." [2]

Four Goals of Life

Ayurveda and Yoga developed during a cultural period of India's history that was broad in its perspective of the significance of human existence. While Yoga developed over a 4,000 year history before being written down as the Yoga Sutras by the sage Patanjali during the time period between 200 BC and the third century, it is suspected that Ayurveda also enjoyed a long history of medical and health studies before being written as the Caraka Samhita towards the end of the first millennium. The prime directive of this culture is to lead a fulfilling life. According to the teachings of Classical India, called the Sanatana Dharma, there are four avenues which must be fulfilled in order to live a full life: dharma (righteous duties); kama (sensual pleasures); artha (material prosperity); and moksha (self-liberation). [3] This way of life requires one to perform duties in a virtuous manner, to maintain the health and vitality necessary to fulfill one's desires, to acquire and possess the material wealth necessary for social position, and the pursuit of peace of mind and spiritual liberation.

For most people, these form a hierarchy of concerns, and accordingly, their pursuit of happiness will be determined by the priority they place on these four avenues. For the Ayurvedic practitioner, the goal is to balance the subtle elements (doshas) so that health may be maintained or restored. For the Yogi, the objective is to promote the spiritual progress of the individual through deepening sadhana as the means to moksha (liberation).

Often, people joke about how difficult life can be, as we were never given an owner's manual for self-care. Ayurveda provides just such an "owner's manual" by presenting us with timeless teachings that inform our decisions for a more fulfilling lifestyle. In contrast, Classical Yoga helps by providing us with detailed guidelines on freeing the positive potentials of the mind for living a fulfilling spiritual life.

Ayurveda and Yoga's Triple Forces

The Yogi's aim is to bring the primal qualities of the three gunas to equilibrium and then to promote the state of spiritual balance that is called harmony or sattva guna. For the Ayurvedic practitioner, the goal is to balance the three qualities called the doshas (fundamental element combinations of ether/air, fire/water, water/earth as they manifest in the visible world) which are seen as the primary driving forces in maintaining and creating health and well-being.

Both Ayurveda and Yoga are based upon the profound study of the forces of life. Their teachings are inter-related, based upon experiences gained through samadhi or deep absorption of the mind into the unchangeable spiritual essence veiled by the diversity of forms. This interrelationship will be made clearer as we discuss the underlying elements of Ayurveda and Yoga. For Ayurveda, these are the doshas, which describe how the building blocks of life are unstable yet follow certain specific patterns. For Yoga, these are the gunas, which are more primal qualities or "threads" that regulate subtler realms to control the direction of all life activities.

In Yoga and Ayurveda, the universe is seen as manifesting three fundamental biological properties. The first property possesses creativity that expresses itself as movement in which the elements air and space are predominant. In Ayurveda, this property is called Vata. In yogic literature, this same biological property is refined into its higher subtler form of energy called prana, which governs rhythm, motion, and sensitivity of the mind. The second property is transformation, which expresses itself as energy or vitality through the elements of fire and water, called Pitta in Ayurveda. Tejas is a refined form of Pitta that creates discernment, the higher function of mind composed of the essence of light. The third property is preservation, which expresses nourishment through the elements of water and earth, called Kapha. Ojas is the refined form of Kapha, providing the foundation of all nurturing qualities that become the immune system, breast milk and the placenta.

The Ayurvedic practitioner learns to feel the life force in food and, in fact, in all manifestations of the material world. He or she comes to know what possesses full potential for health and what doesn't. Lacking or overabundant energy of a dosha is experienced directly; this knowledge is not merely textbook theory. For example, a lack of Vata would be directly experienced as excessive moisture while an overabundance of Vata would be experienced as dryness – raw foods (which will increase Vata) not consumed enough will increase mucous while in overabundance

will increase dryness. The information conveyed by an expert Ayurvedic practitioner is not merely one more alternative method to be free of diseases. By learning
to read the digestive process, the manner in which the quality of food becomes the
skin, facial expressions, tone and pitch of the voice, observe the changes in respiration, reading the twelve radial pulses, and other diagnostic skills, the Ayurvedic
practitioner gains a way to perceive manifestations of life force changes which
are instantaneous. Food is the primal substance from which the body is created,
nurtured, and ultimately, will dissolve into. By studying the changes that life makes
in food, the Ayurvedic practitioner must become a student of the Life Force itself;
only then will the full potential of Ayurveda's scope make itself known.

The entire world manifests in a multiplicity of ways that can be seen through
this worldview or Darshan. Darshan is given in six classical worldviews of which
Patanjali's Yoga Sutras is one. By reading Patanjali's text, we begin to look at the
world through his eyes. His perspective begins to reveal the fullness of life. There is
a tendency for those without a spiritual perspective to see the world as filled with
stagnation, emptiness, or illusion. In contrast, for those with a strong faith in their
world view, the world becomes alive pulsating with the rhythm of life.

The Darshan of Ayurveda shows us how changes in diet, lifestyle, exercise, and
the spiritual practices of Yoga promote health and longevity. Ayurveda directs us
to live a life of fulfillment as stated in Caraka Samhita section entitled Sutrastanam,
chapter I, sutra 55. "The body and mind constitute the substrata of diseases and
happiness [i.e., positive health]. Balanced utilization [of time, mental faculties, and
the objects of sense organs] is the cause of happiness."[4]

Within his own body, the Yogi directly experiences the subtle forces known as
the Ayurvedic doshas. Through this personal experience, the underlying teachings
of the timeless classic, the Yoga Darshan of Patanjali, come to life. It is directly
revealed that the Spiritual Nature of all life becomes known through the disciplines
of yoga that provide the experience of yogic samadhi as the Science of Communion. By sincere practice of Classical Yoga and Ayurveda, a life of service to others
is lived fully. From the inner practices of sustaining harmony with the Life Force
itself, arises the motivation to be of service to all.

The Primal Qualities – The Gunas

For the Yogi, the means to the goal of health, or to "living ones own Self" is
to become "freed from the primordial forces of suffering." [5] In Sanskrit, these
forces arise from the gunas. The gunas are three naturally arising forces. They are
philosophical concepts of the mind. These three states are called tamas, rajas, and
sattva.

The state of balance or harmony is called sattva. This is the goal of yoga therapy
– to achieve a sattvic state of peace and tranquility. For the yogi, it is a naturally
arising state originating from being true to your inner teacher, guru or God. By

purifying the body, senses, and mind, the yogi experiences his natural self.

Individuals tend to identify themselves with their actions, their roles in life, or the praise received from others. This state of activity and hyperactivity is called rajas. It is a mental state in which someone identifies himself with his actions and seeks to gain the rewards of a full life. In the rajasic state, the mind is identified with the concepts of karma, as expressed in the saying that "whatever you sow, you will reap."

The third guna is called tamas. Tamas refers to the darkness, ignorance and lazy nature of the mind or body. This is the force that tells us to take a break and relax when we are near to completing a project whose deadline is approaching. As a result, we do not finish the race. This is similar to the story of the hare and the tortoise. The hare manifested tamasic behavior thinking he was so far ahead of the tortoise that he could sleep, when in fact his sleep led to losing the race. To change this state is to move towards the center of the cycle of the mind – the state of sattva – wherein dwells the True Self.

rajas - sattva - tamas
activity - harmony - inertia

The method recommended to achieve sattva – a balanced state of body and mind in harmony with the natural rhythm of life – is to watch the indicators of balance and carefully adjust lifestyle, diet, physical and mental exercise accordingly. This includes

(1) eating foods which are in season, adopting a vegetarian diet consisting primarily of locally-produced foods;
(2) living a lifestyle in harmony with the seasons so that sleeping, meals and work are regulated daily events;
(3) incorporating meditation and prayer as the first and last events of the day; and
(4) waking and rising before the sun to capture the delight of the glorious sunrise.

In addition, exercise is best during the period before breakfast, followed by a light meal. The major meal of the day would be lunch between 10 a.m. and 2 p.m. The evening meal should be at the time of sunset. The hour prior to bedtime can be spent in restful and pleasant activity such as reading or a walk in nature with bedtime around 10 p.m. and not later than 11 p.m.

The Three Doshas

In Ayurveda, five basic elements of creation - earth, water, fire, air, and ether - manifest as the three biological energy forces, called the doshas. These three qualities are: Vata composed of air and ether; Pitta composed of fire and water; and Kapha composed of earth and water. The three doshas can be seen as the vitalizing forces of life; when they are in balance, health and clarity are the natural outcome. Frawley's <u>Ayurvedic Healing</u> defines dosha as "that which darkens, spoils, or causes things to decay." It implies that which is unstable. When out of balance, the doshas cause disease, decay and death - this is their nature. If we are to make full use of the limited lifespan we are given, it is important to understand these principles and balance our lifestyle to minimize the negative effects of the doshas.

Each individual is composed of a mixture of the doshas. "It is important to remember that these descriptions reflect the pure aspect of each constitutional element: however, no individual constitution is made up solely of any one element. Rather, each person is a combination of all three elements, with a predominant tendency toward one or more." [6] The seven resulting combination of doshas that exist are: Vata predominant (Vata/Pitta, Vata/Kapha, Vata/Pitta/Kapha); Pitta predominant (Pitta/Vata, Pitta/Kapha); and Kapha predominant (Kapha/Pitta, Kapha/Vata).

Koshas: The Subtle Bodies

The yogic perspective of anatomy is quite different from that of Western anatomy. In the yogic view (Darshan) we are composed of five bodies (Pancha Maya koshas). The first body is the same in both yogic and Western views, but the other four bodies are unique to the yogic Darshan. The names of these bodies reveal a radically different perception of reality. In the second chapter of the <u>Taittiriya Upanishad</u>, it is said that our true nature is hidden from our perception because five sheaths enclose it. Each of these sheaths has their own language and method of communicating amongst the layers of the personality.

The first yoga body is called the Annamaya Kosha, literally the "body sheath made of food, which is an illusion." This is our physical body. The physical body is created by and sustained by food. If the quality of the food is high, the illusory nature of the body is more readily perceived. This is one reason why live, fresh, seasonal food from vegetables and fruits is recommended as a yogic diet. Eating fresh food prepared immediately before eating, results in an increase in live vitality available to nurture this "food body." When we eat overcooked foods, stale foods, or animals the food body becomes de-vitalized and has difficulty refining the food to a quality necessary to be converted into the needs of the second body.

The second body is hidden by a subtler sheath and is called the Pranamaya Kosha, the "body sheath made of prana, which is an illusion." This subtle body's anatomy is made of energy channels called nadis, which terminate in spinning energy centers called chakras. The word chakra means wheel, implying an ever-spinning center of activity. The subtle body is composed of our senses and emotional states. The energy flowing through these channels is sensory input from the five gross senses and the subtler senses associated with the mind. Hence these vortices and channels are always active during our waking state seeking sensory and emotional stimulation. When we are fed beautiful sense impressions - art, nature, live vibrant colorful aromatic food - they can be converted into the "prana" which keeps this subtle body healthy. From these stimuli, the chakras become open and functional. When we are not interested, repulsed or fall asleep, the chakras activity slows down or stops. The energies withdraw from the outer world and become replenished provided they can assimilate the sensory input provided. With negative input - violent movies, stale odors, and chemical food - there is less vitality available to be converted to prana.

The third body is called the Manomaya Kosha, the "body sheath made of thought, which is an illusion." This is the body of the mind. This body is made up of the refinements produced from the first two bodies as well as its own capacity to generate positive uplifting thoughts. When thoughts are beneficial, the mind is content and at peace. From this, more positivity is generated and the mind refreshes itself. The nature of this body is thought. Mantra can transform the mind to a higher level of perception and cognition. Mantra literally means "the word which when contemplated transforms the mind." Mantras given properly as a meal prepared lovingly will plug the mind into a higher and more creative mind, which thinks of the welfare of others.

The fourth body is the Vijnanamaya Kosha, the "body sheath made of wisdom, which is an illusion." This body is made of transcendent thoughts. It is awareness that is free of self-centeredness. It is concerned for the welfare of all. This is generated by a naturally-arising state of detachment from the grosser bodies. This body knows it is not the physical food body; therefore, one established in this awareness is indifferent to what happens to the body. For what happens to the physical body does not change the state of wisdom. Wisdom is the beginning of contact with transcendence. This state is accessed by meditation, reflection, and giving it proper food. The proper food is good company, spiritual literature, and selfless service to others. By a regular diet of these nutritious foods, the body of wisdom becomes more active and can fend off periods of unwholesome contact.

The fifth body is the Anandamaya Kosha, the "body sheath of bliss, which is also an illusion." This body is said to be as small as a mustard seed, seated in the secret chamber of the interior heart to the right of the physical heart. This body is composed of happiness. It does not need anything to generate its happiness, as that is its natural state. The beneficial foods given to the four grosser bodies will be refined into the food, which makes up this body. But also it is by nature joyful. And that is not the end. According to the Yoga Philosophy there is hidden beyond this body the Truth of Who you are.

Each of the bodies hides the next one. And yet it also reveals something of the subtler body. The physical body appears to possess energy and vitality and yet it derives that substance from the subtler body of prana. In turn, when we have energy and emotional fulfillment, our mind appears healthy yet it derives mind substance from yet a subtler source.

This is how yogis perceive health. This process proceeds from the grosser kosha being fulfilled then it naturally produces a refined energy that becomes the material of the subtler kosha. Thus, health of the body produces a by-product which is vitality and emotional health. This creates a tendency for mental health. If the higher koshas are dis-eased by negative thinking or emotions they will block the efforts of the more gross koshas toward health. Hence, energy becomes wasted and the student's attainments are unstable. Classical Yoga is more concerned with the relationship of the third and fourth koshas bringing the mind into a receptive mode with the source of higher knowledge. All the Yoga sadhanas (practices to establish a spiritual lifestyle) seek to promote health and the full receptivity of the being to the Creative Spirit.

And so for the yogi, health is not merely determined by the physical body, nor is it created by physical exercise alone. The Sanskrit word for health is svastha, which literally translated means "established in the Self." To the yogis, true health is a coming home to your Self. In the condition of not being at home to your Self, there is dis-ease.

Yoga Refined: The Five Prana Vayus

The principle element that the Yogi focuses upon is prana, experienced as the first of the four subtle bodies, the Pranamaya Kosha. This quality is what is sought during the practice of asana. For it is from maintaining a regular disciplined lifestyle and physical manipulations that the yogi creates more prana and the ability to sustain it within himself. One of the definitions of a yogi that I like is that a yogi is one whose prana does not leave their body. By following the guidelines of Patanjali's Yoga Sutras on asana and pranayama in chapter II, 46-53 one gradually develops the lifting of the veil that "obscures the radiant supreme light of the inner Self" [7] These sutras describe the process of naturally-arising experiences that progressively lead to freeing the mind of its false perceptions of reality.

In the ancient Hindu texts, the life force was called a Vayu, meaning wind or air. The more contemporary treatises call the life force prana. Prana is seen as the intermediary force behind the mind, the force that creates movement in all arenas of life. Its subtlest component is the movement of thought. So as we regulate the prana we can slow down the speed of thought and direct it toward a specific task. There are five Pranas (Prana, Samana, Udana, Apana, and Vyana), all of which are subdivisions of Vata.

The first and primary prana is more properly called Adya Prana. In its universal or primary form, this force is omnipresent, it is said to be "that which is everywhere at all times." As it moves within the human body, prana, literally the "forward moving air" or the "in breath," descends into the chest region from the nostrils, progressing downward and inward as the inhalation.

Samana, the "mid-breath" or the "balancing air," moves from the outer body to the center and serves to absorb beneficial material. In the respiratory cycle, it is active during the pause following the inhalation. It is especially located in the abdominal organs and centered in the small intestine.

Udana, the "upward moving air," moves upward as the first portion of the exhalation. Udana moves opposite of Prana as it is responsible for moving our attention outward into the universe. It primarily resides in the chest cavity, though when balanced it is centered in the trachea where it governs speech and exhalation.

Apana, the "out-breath" or "the air that moves away," is the prana that moves downward and outward functioning as the last portion of the exhalation. As it leaves the body, it is experienced as warmer than the inhaled air. It predominates in the lower abdomen and is centered in the pelvic cavity (located at the bottom of the pelvis). It governs movements from the navel down to rectum and from the hips to the feet. This prana is concentrated in those organs that separate and eliminate waste products of menstrual fluids, urine, and feces.

Vyana, the "through-breath" or the "outward moving air," moves from the body's center and sends vitality to the peripheral regions of the body. It governs movements from the navel throughout the body. It governs the heart and circulation to all levels of the mind/body. Its basic dynamic is as a centrifugal force. Vyana Prana maintains the voluntary muscles and skeletal system for conscious motions and is responsible for involuntary movements that maintain health of these systems.

When perfect health is present, this pranic cycle feeds each of the pranas in turn and they create health. Health is a multidimensional concept; similarly the pranas affect the different koshas generating health when consciousness is permitted to return to its source as the inner Self.

A Yogic Perspective on Ayurveda

Dr. Vasant Lad, a foremost exponent of Ayurveda, has said that Ayurveda and Yoga are sister sciences, implying that they share a similar worldview and descended from the same root. Yet these sisters are clearly not twins; they take different directions in fulfilling their objectives. From my perspective, Ayurvedic teachings provide the foundation for physical health and Yoga develops our spiritual side. When they are carefully studied and developed into a personal lifestyle through guidance from an experienced teacher, these practices lead to a harmonious personality.

As a Yogi, my perspective is that all my clients are spiritual seekers whether they declare themselves to be or not. My intention is to help them live a lifestyle that gives the experience of this doshic evolution of Vata, Pitta, and Kapha into their higher manifestations as peace, discriminative insight, and love. My goal is to stabilize and enrich the foundational positive qualities of the balanced doshas.

I prioritize my attention according to the state of the five bodies (Pancha Maya koshas), paying less attention to the vacillations (vrittis) of physical health relating to the gross body; more attention to balance of the five pranas of the subtle body; and even more attention to the generating of positive thoughts for health of the mental body. I strive to share how to nurture their most subtle bodies – the bodies of wisdom and bliss through spiritual practices and keeping good, uplifting company both inwardly and socially.

When this is accomplished, the student, through the evolution of their Vata qualities, is able to touch their intuitive source and that increased prana guides them in the form of their inner teacher. Their Pitta qualities induce discernment and the experience of knowing the mind's root as the source of spiritual light. Finally their Kapha quality can evolve into compassion and open-heartedness, thereby increasing their capacity for love and nurturance of the Self, and that blessing is naturally extended to all beings.

It is often unclear in Ayurvedic teachings whether there is a need to increase, or decrease the dosha that is imbalanced; for this reason the person may have a prescribed practice very different from another. There are three major models for working with Ayurvedic principles to restore harmony. In the most prevalent approach, an Ayurvedic practitioner strives to decrease the qualities of a dosha that has been elevated. This striving to achieve balance is an ongoing practice (sadhana).

In the second, one increases the opposite quality in a different dosha. This is the method for relieving the primary attributes of each dosha as described in one of the original treatises on Ayurveda, the Caraka Samhita. [8] For example, when working with an elevated Kapha as manifested by increased lethargy, one might choose rigorous, heat increasing practice such as Bikram or Ashtanga Yoga, which would elevate Pitta and makes them detoxify by sweating.

Finally, a third approach is to focus attention to doing Yogasanas resulting in a balanced state of the dosha. Thus positive attributes such as strength, stamina, patience, open heart, and humility will predominate. The practices would differ based upon whether Kapha was imbalanced due to rajas (hyperactivity) or tamas (lethargy). For rajasic Kapha, in which the student is overactive in their physical health maintenance, I would have the student hold the posture to develop patience and perseverance while relaxing their overactive efforts. They need to read and reflect on Yoga Sutras II, 47. For tamasic Kapha, the student would be encouraged to push themselves with the resulting warmth directed not merely at overcoming lethargy but at opening their heart. They need to reflect on Yoga Sutras II, 48 and begin to seek the experience of duality and its opposite. The goal is to achieve a balanced or sattvic experience of Kapha and then elevate that to produce ojas, the experience that can lead to the states of joy and love (anandamayaAnandamaya kosha). This is my preferred way of working with students.

In applying this third approach to imbalanced Vata, note that rajasic Vata students will tend to move too much. They will not be able to be still for long and often can be seen squirming in between instructions in yoga class. They need to watch their pranic currents and not immediately react to them, being sensitive yet not reactive. They need to read and be reminded of Yoga Sutras I, 30-31. For tamasic Vata, they will be the opposite and not listen to what the teacher is saying. They will follow their own inner voice and become lost in the maze of mind. There is frequently an indication of them entering into a realm of fascination but not one of elevation. They need to reflect on Yoga Sutras II, 1-11 and seek practical advice on how to manifest these teachings.

The rajasic Pitta will continue to focus on the "burn" on being stimulated and hot. Their practice will feed their desire for stimulation yet will lack discernment about how much effort to do or how much is too hot. They need to read Yoga Sutras II, 40-41 and also 46 and see that these are important building blocks to attaining self mastery that they seek so adamantly. The tamasic Pitta will be afraid of their energy and power thus developing into lethargy mentally and physically. While the same sutras will apply to them, they also need to reflect on Yoga Sutras II, 42-43 for without freedom from impurities the contentment that they are truly seeking will remain a fantasy.

To reestablish sattvic state all practices need to follow the Classical Yoga guidelines and seek the tried and proven path to harmony. It is not so much the technique that is at fault; it is the problem with the attitude, intention, and force with which the techniques are applied. When the student is not clear about the intention of the practice, they will be guided by their perception of their imbalance du jour. Such shortsightedness is characteristic of a Vata imbalance. The greatest way to restore balance is finding a teacher of depth and seeking their advice.

The major pranayama needed for restoring Kapha to a sattvic state is Kapalabhati taught as one of the six purifying actions (Shatkarma Kriya). When taught for the purpose of purifying Kapha, it can keep the tendency of Kapha, which is to congeal into tightness and excessive mucous, to a minimum. This pranayama can be beneficial for all major Kapha disorders when taught by teachers who are adept at its usage for themselves. It promotes courage, hopefulness, faithfulness, and humility. These are natural qualities that come from an increase in ojas. On the physical level ojas represents health and the strength of the immune system. For the Yogi, ojas is the love of the Self as God within, the capacity to love and accept all as unique aspects of the singular Divinity. The pranayamas for each dosha will be given in detail in chapter 14 entitled "Ayurvedic Yoga Therapy – Dosha Balancing."

I am not too concerned with the maintenance of health via balancing the doshas if spiritual practice, sadhana, is thereby compromised. What is the result of good spiritual practice – peace is the sign Vata is balanced and sattvic; enthusiasm and love of life is Pitta balanced; and love and understanding of others is a sattvic Kapha experience. Of course, during sadhana the barriers to these balanced states will naturally arise to find their way out. During this process of Kriya Yoga in which impurities of body, prana, negative emotions and thoughts are removed, the student is likely to be uncomfortable and may not take care of his or her body. One may stay up too late processing all that is arising, have a binge of eating comfort foods, or may overly indulge in sensual pleasures. All these will have a negative impact on health, but in the long run when commitment to sadhana is secured, such events are minor bumps in the spiritual path.

This attitude is disturbing to some health practitioners who seek physical health. I perceive the challenges brought upon by a temporary period of strong spiritual practice as necessary and ultimately beneficial disturbances leading toward greater alignment with the guidance of Spirit. My intention is to bring consciousness to reflect upon the relative importance of health as contrasted with spirituality. What is the primary interest the student has? The confusion between the four goals of life has led to many twists on one's karmic path. From the Yogic perspective, righteous duty (dharma) is naturally carried out by practicing the first two of the eight limbs (Ashtanga) of Classical Yoga, the ten ethics of yama and niyama. Those who live a righteous life will experience the movement towards the attainments that are cited by Patanjali in chapter II, 35-45. For instance, "By abiding in truthfulness, one's words and actions are subservient to truth and thus whatever is said or done bears the fruit of that sincerity." [9] Living from this foundation, life will naturally produce pleasure and abundance (kamaKama and artha). There is no need to do separate practices for their fulfillment.

As most serious seekers know, doing sadhana with sincerity and devotion can imbalance the doshas since it is seeking to remove the obstructive patterns laid down by years or even lifetimes of fixed mental attitudes and behaviors. This is most pronounced in those seekers who have had a spiritual awakening. Kundalini is the latent spiritual energy most commonly awakened by manipulating Udana prana. It can become temporarily awakened via willful practices like sustained back bending asanas, long rajasic practice of energetic breathing exercises (pranayama), austere dieting and fasting, and mantras. These types of awakening are short lived and often produce tremendous imbalances in the mental and physical aspects of the doshas. A knowledgeable Ayurvedic practitioner can be of help to restore them to serenity.

Students who lack experienced guidance often pursue these practices subconsciously motivated by a desire for success in any of the other goals of life, rather than a sincere desire for spiritual liberation. They must suffer the consequences of their misdirected actions. However in true spiritual awakening, which comes from Spirit seeking to know its own nature, the imbalances of the doshas that arise are more like a flowering of a preexisting condition. They are relatively easy to overcome when following the guidance of a spiritual guide whose devotional foundation is solid.

The great revolutionary philosopher Sri Aurobindo said "Yoga is condensed evolution." The Yogini experiencing spiritual awakening begins to sense that she is moving through lifetimes within her one current lifetime. To become successful in fulfilling the goal of spiritual liberation (moksha), the seeker is encouraged to develop a relationship with the body based on personalizing the teachings with discrimination, "detachment and consistent earnest effort" as described in the Yoga Sutras I, 12.

Certainly one can utilize Yogasanas to help maintain balance in the unstable doshas, yet the Yogini knows better than to put all her attention into health maintenance. The concern for health is balanced with the need for purification in the opening aphorism of chapter two of Patanjali's Yoga Sutras. "This sutra describes the threefold process of Kriya Yoga necessary to prepare the mind for the experience of yoga. It consists of self-study (svadhyaya) that correlates in Ayurvedic language to a deeply pacifying method for balancing Vata, which develops the prana, and stilling the mind. The second component is self-discipline and purification (tapas) corresponding to Pitta practice for strengthening and directing willpower. The third component is devotion to God (Isvara-pranidhana), which fulfills the deepest desire of the Kapha dosha for a lifelong pursuit of selfless service. When studied together Ayurveda and Classical Yoga have tremendous potential for speeding up the course of one's maturity." [10]

II. Ayurvedic Concepts

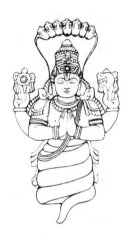

The Twenty Attributes of the Doshas

The three primal qualities of Nature, the gunas, manifest as three forces, according to the <u>Caraka Samhita</u>, Sutrastanam I, 49. The first category consists of the five elements – earth, water, fire, air, and ether – as they manifest as smell, taste, vision, touch, and sound, respectively); the second is the 20 attributes; and the third relates to the soul, including qualities such as the intellect, memory, consciousness, ego, virtues, and discernment.

The twenty attributes are divided into ten pairs of opposites. Their properties are manifest throughout nature and give us the ability to define and structure the world within and around us. By understanding and perceiving each of these attributes, we can comprehend the current state of affairs as well as the direction of change from the point of balance or sattva. As you read the list, consider an experience of each of them that you have recently had. By contrasting the polar opposites of the attributes, you can come to know the immediacy of change that they can create.

1. Cold – Hot
2. Wet - Dry
3. Heavy - Light
4. Gross – Subtle
5. Dense – Flowing
6. Static – Mobile
7. Dull – Sharp
8. Soft – Hard
9. Smooth – Rough
10. Cloudy – Clear

Comprehension of the attributes helps us to understand the primal changes that take place within and around us all the time. Subtle changes within the body and breath are occurring each moment, but without the capacity to sense them, we can be overcome by the volatility of a turbulent mind. Without a sattvic mental state, this turbulence creates anxiety and disturbed thinking. Questions arise in the mind that can have no easy answer: How did I get here? Why does this keep happening to me? What's going to happen to me? Why Me?

By cultivating a sattvic attitude, questions that stimulate creativity and that can have beneficial answers can arise. How can I improve my relationships? How can I be of more loving service to others? What can I do to improve my conscious contact with Spirit on a moment-to-moment basis?

An examination of the attributes of your body or breath will assist you in comprehending your changes to the environment, which in turn will assist you in becoming self aware, though not necessarily more comfortable initially. But in the long run, this will enable you to adapt to change without stress. It is this ability to adapt that Ayurveda and Yoga seek to promote. By knowing your own constitution and the qualities of the objects of your senses, you can predict how you will likely respond. With patience and perseverance, you can learn to prepare yourself for predictable changes of the seasons or changes in life that are foreseeable. By making Yoga and Ayurveda into a lifestyle, you will increase your capacity to ride the waves of life's current.

The qualities of the ten pairs of opposites in relationship to the doshas

1. Hot is most associated with the element fire and the dosha Pitta.
    ⬆ P   ⬇ K & V
    Cold is associated with all the elements except fire. The gross elements of earth and water retain heat, while the subtle elements of air and ether disperse it.
    ⬆ K & V   ⬇ P
2. Wet is most associated with water and Kapha.
    ⬆ K (mildly P)   ⬇ V
    Dry is an air quality related to Vata. All the elements are dry except water. Earth can hold water while the other elements tend to disperse it.
    ⬆ V   ⬇ K (mildly P)
3. Heavy is especially associated with earth and water elements. It strongly diminishes Vata and moderately diminishes Pitta.
    ⬆ K   ⬇ V & P
    Light relates to fire, air and ether.
    ⬆ V & P   ⬇ K
4. Gross is associated with earth and water. It strongly diminishes Vata and moderately diminishes Pitta.
    ⬆ K   ⬇ V & P
    Subtle is related to fire, air and ether. It strongly increases Vata and moderately increases Pitta.
    ⬆ V & P   ⬇ K
5. Dense relates to the earth.
    ⬆ K   ⬇ V & P
    Flowing or liquidrelates to water and fire. It moderately decreases Kapha and strongly decreases Vata.
    ⬆ P   ⬇ V & K
6. Mobile (sometimes thought of as fast) is a quality of both air and fire. It strongly increases Vata and moderately increases Pitta.
    ⬆ V & P   ⬇ K
    Static (considered as slow) is the quality of earth and water. Strongly decreases Vata and moderately decreases Pitta.
    ⬆ K   ⬇ V & P

7. Dull is the quality of earth and water. It strongly decreases Vata and moderately decreases Pitta.

   ↑ K   ↓ V & P

   Sharp or penetrating relates to fire, air and ether. Fire is the sharpest of substances. It strongly increases Pitta and moderately increases Vata.

   ↑ P & V   ↓ K

8. Soft is the quality of water. It strongly increases Kapha, moderately increases Pitta, and strongly decreases Vata.

   ↑ K & P   ↓ V

   Hard is the qualities of air and earth. It strongly increases Kapha and Vata, mildly decreases Pitta.

   ↑ V & K   ↓ P

9. Smooth is a quality of water. It strongly increases Kapha, moderately increases Pitta, and strongly diminishes Vata.

   ↑ K & P   ↓ V

   Rough is a quality associated with air and earth. It increases Vata, strongly diminishes Kapha, and moderately decreases Pitta.

   ↑ V   ↓ P & K

10. Clear or light relates to fire, air, and ether. It strongly increases Vata, moderately increases Pitta, and decreases Kapha

    ↑ V & P   ↓ K

    Cloudy or dark relates to earth and water.

    ↑ K   ↓ V & P

Summary of the Attributes

Cold/hot, wet/dry, heavy/light, gross/subtle, dense/flowing, static/mobile, dull/sharp, soft/hard, smooth/rough, cloudy, clear

Vata – cold, dry, light, subtle, flowing, mobile, sharp, hard, rough, clear
Pitta – hot, slightly wet, light, subtle, flowing, mobile, sharp, soft, smooth, clear
Kapha – cold, wet, heavy, gross, dense, static, dull, soft, smooth, cloudy

Both Vata and Pitta share the attributes of light, subtle, mobile, sharp, and clear. Kapha and Pitta have in common the attributes of wet, liquid, soft, and smooth. Vata and Kapha have in common only the attribute of cold.

In Ayurvedic pulse diagnosis, the doshas are experienced as resembling the motions of three animals. Pitta is in continuous motion like a snake; Vata is disconnected with pauses like a frog jumping. Kapha is smooth, balanced motions likened to graceful motions of a swan on a calm lake.

Earth and water combine to form the Kapha dosha. Water and fire combine to form the Pitta dosha. Air and ether combine to form the Vata dosha.

We are all born with an inherent constitutional balance of these three doshas.

When they are in balance, they create a state of physical and psychological harmony, an experience of Yoga. When imbalanced, they create a sense of dis-ease.

Ether – cold, dry, light, subtle, liquid, mobile, sharp, soft, smooth, clear
Air – cold, dry, light, subtle, mobile, sharp, rough, hard, clear
Fire – hot, dry, light, subtle, mobile, sharp, rough, hard, clear
Water – cold, wet, heavy, gross, liquid, static, dull, soft, smooth, cloudy
Earth – cold, dry, heavy, gross, solid, static, dull, hard, rough, cloudy

Vata – The Principle of Motion

Vata is the combination of air and ether elements with air predominating over ether. The word Vata means "that which moves." "Vata is the principle of movement in the body and the energy that governs biological movement in the body. . . . Vata regulates breathing, all movements of the muscles and tissues, the heart muscle, and all biological movements, intracellular and extra cellular, including the single movements of the nerve impulses."[11] It brings substances into the body, transports them to their beneficial sites for metabolism, and expels waste products from the tissues. It governs all life functions and manifests as the life force called Prana. The Yogic term Prana, and the more ancient term Vayu, are synonymous with the Ayurvedic term Vata. In the mind, it creates peace, open-mindedness, adaptability, intuition, and a higher intelligence concerned with Oneness. Vata governs the region from the waist down. Its home neighborhood is the pelvic cavity. It's seat of balance is the colon.

While Vata's principle function is to create motion, it also includes the primary characteristics from the twenty attributes of cold, dry, light, subtle, mobile, sharp, hard, rough, and clear. This is the most important of the doshas, for changes in it occur before all others. Bringing it to balance restores the system. Vata is divided into five functional forms – Prana, Udana, Samana, Apana, and Vyana. These are the same in Yogic and Ayurvedic literature.

Prana as the first subtype of Vata is more properly called Adya Prana, the primary prana. It governs intake and moves down from the head into the chest. In an imbalanced state, it is the root source of all disease and pain. It especially creates respiratory disorders, mental problems, neurological disorders and difficulties of the head, specifically the brain.

Udana Prana governs output and moves upward from the chest toward the head. In a spiritually-developed individual, Udana becomes elevated and transformed then renamed as Kundalini Shakti. Signs of this elevation are experiences of spiritual awakening, the direct knowledge of a higher power. On a biological level, Udana prana is responsible for diseases of the ears, nose, throat, speech problems, and diseases of the chest.

Samana Prana governs absorption. It rules the region of the abdomen and moves outward from there, spreading nutrients into the tissues throughout the body. It is involved in digestive problems, especially weak or irregular digestion, improper formation of tissues, anorexia, and diarrhea. It rules the liver, spleen, stomach, pancreas, and the upper section of the colon.

Apana Prana governs elimination. Its major motion is downward and outward thus creating excretion of waste through urine, feces and also the release that is sexual climax. With dysfunction, it creates constipation, menstrual problems, sexual dysfunctions, and problems with immunity.

Vyana Prana is the subtlest form of Vata and it rules circulation. It is connected with all diseases, especially circulatory problems, coldness of the extremities and motor problems. It is the subtle energy we call the aura.

In Yoga, we have practices for balancing our Vata qualities to promote natural biological rhythms like menstruation, sleep, and digestion, as well as practices to calm the mind, clarify perceptions, and elevate intuition. On the therapeutic level, these practices are used for osteoarthritis, motion sickness, poor circulation, hypoglycemia, epilepsy, and stress-generated diseases like hypertension, headaches, constipation, and insomnia. Psychologically, they can be adapted to address fear, anxiety, fatigue, self-confidence, improve memory, and to develop a stronger will power. My guru, Swami Muktananda, said that "If the body is weak, Prana flows in and out. When this is the case how can you find any joy in life?"[12]

Ayurveda works by calming the agitated dosha, restoring balance and returning the dosha to its home site. For instance, if Vata is aggravated, it may produce symptoms in different sites such as constipation, dull pain, dry cough, headache, and restlessness. While the doshas have their main region and home organ, they are all pervasive throughout the body. Each dosha produces symptoms that can be in any organ or tissue. Regardless of which dosha is imbalanced, balancing Vata and returning the pranas to their home region and function can rectify all other doshas. For this reason, all students need to have a sadhana that begins and concludes with Vata balancing.

Pitta – the Principle of Transformation

Pitta is the combination of fire and water, with fire as the predominant quality of this dosha. Pitta translates as "that which digests." Its qualities are hot, penetrating, light, mobile, liquid, and slightly oily. Its most characteristic quality is that of transformation. It is most readily apparent as the energy creating body heat. Those persons who are seemingly unaffected by winter's cold and wear T-shirts year round have strong Pitta in their constitution. It gives hair a natural luster and provides subtle oil to the skin to regulate body temperature. It is responsible for all chemical, metabolic reactions including those of the psyche. Pitta imparts the necessary heat for the individual's constitution and regulates metabolic transformations to keep up the radiance of the body. Pitta not only nourishes, it also senses the breakdown of tissues as they are transformed back into waste material (ama). Ama is a malfunctioning digestive problem. It represents undigested food and the waste tissues formed as feces, urine and sweat. Pitta regulates the cycle rotating between nourishment and waste.

Pitta manifests as our hunger and thirst to stimulate and provide nourishment. Diminished Pitta is common as we age, and with it, a loss of the sense of thirst. Subtle signals of thirst must be retrained and cultivated. Thirst must be re-established to balance metabolism. This requires reminding oneself to drink frequently until the thirst reflex begins to naturally assert itself. In people over 40 this may take two months or more.

Pitta allows material and information to be changed into substances that are beneficial for the Life Force. It digests information and changes it into experiences and data that we can utilize. It governs digestion, assimilation, and nutrition. In its most subtle form, it manifests as Tejas, the fire that transforms yet nourishes. In the mind, it manifests as enthusiasm, vitality, interest, curiosity and love of life. Pitta governs the region from the diaphragm to the top of the pelvis. Its home neighborhood is the abdominal cavity and its seat of balance is the small intestine.

There are five subtypes of Pitta: Pachaka, Sadhaka, Alochaka, Bhrajaka, and Ranjaka.

Pachaka is the fire of digestion. It is responsible for absorption of nutrients in the small intestine. This is the primary form of Pitta and manifests as the digestive fire known as Agni. It moves similarly to Samana Prana, moving outward, distributing nutrients to our tissues. It also has a discriminating function that separates beneficial nutrients from those that are not healthy. In normal function, it destroys that which is not beneficial.

Sadhaka Pitta is located in the brain and is the light of right understanding and discrimination. Its root "sadh" means "to realize" as the word sadhana means the way to realization. Therefore, this form of Pitta creates the ability of the mind to realize the true Self. It functions on both a worldly level to direct us toward fulfilling personal goals and on the higher level for spiritual development. Similar to the movement of the primary Adya Prana, its primary movement is inward.

Alochaka Pitta is in the eyes and is responsible for visual acuity, perception of depth, color, size, and shape. When functioning well, vision is clear and the eyes are lustrous. In iridology, the science of iris analysis, the clarity of the iris reveals the health of the internal structures. Lack of clarity is seen with darkness or malformations of energy lines within the iris. Like Udana Prana, it moves upward and helps to promote a more spiritual vision of the world.

Bhrajaka Pitta is in the skin, giving it its temperature and color. It promotes absorption through the skin when using mineral waters, medicated oils or medicines applied to the skin. It is the heat that generates perspiration. It generates the warm of the body and promotes the glow we associate with our aura. It moves similarly to Vyana Prana and has an outward motion.

Ranjaka Pitta is in the liver and is responsible for the secondary level of digestion that takes place on the tissue level. It is the form of Pitta that gives color to the blood and waste products. It produces warmth in the blood and circulatory system. It moves similarly to Apana Prana in having a downward motion that can help to expel wastes.

Agni is an interrelated aspect of Pitta. It is the bodily fire that transforms foods into body tissues and information into knowledge and experience. The main site of Agni is in the small intestine. It's name is Jatharagni and it is responsible for the primary level of digestion of food. From here, it feeds the other twelve subtypes of Agni situated throughout the body. If the primary Agni is low, other tissues and the mind suffer from lack of the ability to transform intake into useable products. Therefore, ama or waste products begin to accumulate which can damage the tissues by creating sluggish function, obstruction to the movement of fluids or loss of bodily heat.

The yoga practices for balancing Pitta energy promote a good appetite with strong digestive fire, heighten our enjoyment of life, and maintain the stability of our vitality. Therapeutically, these practices are used for inflammatory conditions such as arthritis, ulcer, colitis, acne, and sciatica. The psychological applications include conditions of anger, excessive self-criticism, dissatisfaction with life, and jealousy.

Kapha – the Principle of Stability

Kapha is the combination of earth and water elements, with water being the primary constituent. The word translates as "that which holds together." Its qualities from the twenty attributes are cold, wet, heavy, gross, static, dull, and cloudy. Kapha governs tissue growth, strength, stability, and natural tissue resistance. It lubricates the joints in the form of synovial fluid, promotes coolness in the intestines and stomach as the mucosal lining, cools the skin as perspiration, gives vitality to the heart and lungs, and helps heal wounds. It governs growth, maintenance, and longevity on the cellular level, and stabilizes the auto-immune system to promote stamina. On the mental level, it promotes qualities such as patience, endurance, calmness, serenity, and devotion. Kapha governs the region from the head to the diaphragm. Its home region is the chest cavity and its seat of balance is the heart.

Kapha manifests in five forms as Avalambaka, Tarpaka, Bodhaka, Kledaka, and Shleshaka.

Avalambaka Kapha is the primary form of Kapha located in the chest, especially in the heart and in the vertebral column. Its name means "that which gives support." It protects the vital organs of the heart and lungs and promotes ease of motion and stamina in the back. It is the storehouse of Kapha and all other forms are governed by its health. For example, clearing the chest of mucous has a longer lasting effect than clearing the symptomatic tissue of its increased Kapha. Avalambaka Kapha moves downward like Apana Prana and gives the feeling of being grounded with emotional and physical stability. When increased too much, it causes major diseases due to over-accumulation of tissue, hardening and excess mucous.

Kledaka Kapha is principally in the stomach as the form that moistens. It protects the stomach lining from the stomach acids and gases of Pachaka Pitta that are necessary for digestion. Thus, it has a discriminating factor in that it protects the stomach yet allows the fire to be strong enough to do its duty. It moves inward like Samana Prana to balance and discern what is beneficial from that which is potentially harmful.

Bodhaka Kapha is in the taste buds and mucous of the mouth. It protects the tissues from foods that are too hot or cold. It is the form that gives perception, especially of taste. Iced beverages and cold foods lessen this and diminish the effectiveness of digestion, which can contribute to slowed metabolism and a tendency for constipation. It moves like Udana Prana upward to promote self-awareness and enjoyment of the senses.

Tarpaka Kapha is in the brain and spinal cord as cerebral spinal fluid (CSF). It protects the brain from injury and also supplies nutrients to the nervous system. It is a form of water that promotes contentment (tripti). On the subtle side, it imparts calmness, happiness, and memory. Its primary motion is inward like Adya Prana and gives the feeling of contentment as arising from within oneself. It builds especially from regularity in meditation.

Shleshaka Kapha is in the joints and protects them from wear, providing smooth function of the skeletal joints. Its name means "that which gives lubrication" (the Sanskrit word "slish" means to be moist and sticky). It is synovial fluid and when healthy prevents arthritis. It moves outward like Vyana Prana regulating strength and stability in joint motions.

Optimal Kapha Balance

Good health is the natural outcome of a balanced Kapha quality. This is the biological goal for the Ayurvedic practitioner. The psychological goal achieved by Kapha balance is compassion and natural charity to help others.

> *"If you haven't any charity in your heart,*
> *you have the worst kind of heart trouble."*
> Bob Hope [13]

For the Yogi, once Kapha is balanced, a veil over consciousness is lifted, revealing the underlying Spirit. The Yogi's process of purification leads to the experiences of the mystic. The great Sufi poet Rumi describes this veil beautifully.

"Between God and his servant are just two veils, all other veils manifest from these two: health and wealth.

He who is healthy says, "Where is God? I don't know and I don't see." As soon as he begins to suffer he says, "Oh God! Oh God!" He begins sharing his secrets with Him and talking to Him. So you see that health was his veil and God was hidden under his pain.

So long as man has riches, he gathers together all the means of achieving his desires. Night and day he busies himself with them. But as soon as he loses his wealth, his ego weakens and he turns round about God."

Rumi, Fihi ma Fihi 233/240.[14]

For the Yogi, the effort is about lifting the veil and experiencing the cosmic dance between God/dess and the Self in its humblest form.

Subdoshas and their Interrelationships

The primary forms of the doshas are as follows:

Adya Prana   Pachaka Pitta   Avalambaka Kapha

The five subdoshas share an interrelationship based on their functions and bodily locations. Below, the first line relates to the brain, heart and nervous system. They are the controllers of the other forms of their subdoshas. The second line is centered in the head and relates to the ability to take in and digest sensory stimulation. The third line relates to the digestive process. The fourth line relates to the surface of the body and the limbs. The last line is the subtlest form of the subdoshas and supports their other functions.

Adya Prana	Sadhaka Pitta	Tarpaka Kapha
Udana Prana	Alochaka Pitta	Bodhaka Kapha
Samana Prana	Pachaka Pitta	Kledaka Kapha
Vyana Prana	Bhrajaka Pitta	Shleshaka Kapha
Apana Prana	Ranjaka Pitta	Avalambaka Kapha

They also share similar motions as follows:

Down and inward	Adya Prana	Sadhaka Pitta	Tarpaka Kapha
Upward	Udana Prana	Alochaka Pitta	Bodhaka Kapha
Circular and inward	Samana Prana	Pachaka Pitta	Kledaka Kapha
Circular and outward	Vyana Prana	Bhrajaka Pitta	Shleshaka Kapha
Down and outward	Apana Prana	Ranjaka Pitta	Avalambaka Kapha

Summary of the Subdoshas

Vata

Subdosha	location	motion	physiology	yoga practices
Adya	Head, chest, heart	Down & in	Senses, nervous system	Ujjaye
Udana	Throat, diaphragm	Upward	Speech, memory	Kapalabhati
Samana	Small intestine	Circular inward	Agni, absorb food	Agnisar dhouti
Vyana	Lymph, joints, heart	Spreading outward	Blood/lymph, circulation	Shatkarmas
Apana	Large intestine	Down & outward	Wastes, sexual fluids	basti

Pitta

Sadhaka	Heart/brain	Understanding	Nadisodhana
Alochaka	Eyes	Vision	Tratak
Pachaka	Small intestine	Digestion	Bhastrika
Bhrajaka	Skin	Luster, body temp.	Danta dhouti
Ranjaka	Liver, spleen	Coloring	dhouti

Kapha

Tarpaka	Head	Pleasing	Absorb shock, cools memory	Tratak, kapalabhati
Bodhaka	Root of tongue	Feeling	Taste, appetite	Neti
Kledaka	Stomach	Moistening	Aids digestion	Basti
Shleshaka	Joints	Lubricating	Smooth motion	Pavanmuktasana
Avalambaka	Lungs, heart	Supporting	Lungs	Vamana dhouti

Ayurvedic Constitutional Body Types

An important concept to keep in mind when considering the basic constitution, or Prakruti, is that the Ayurvedic doshas that create the constitution are biological, i.e., physical qualities. They are not the same as the energies of the yogic subtle body system of the centers (chakras) and channels (nadis), in spite of both possessing elemental (earth, water, fire, air, and ether) qualities.

Everyone has a specific constitution, or Prakruti, comprised of a mixture of the three doshas. Classic Ayurvedic texts also mention a fourth dosha, Sama which is an even mixture of Vata/Pitta/Kapha; but this is extremely rare. Indeed Dr. David Frawley, a preeminent writer on Ayurveda, claims that while this is theoretically possible, he has not seen even one example of a single dosha constitution person. Hence, people manifest as one of the dual or tridoshic constitutions[15] and the Sama dosha is quite rare, though it does exist in theory.

This leaves us with six other combinations of constitution, which we will discover in examining ourselves. The most likely possibilities are all dual constitutions. The most common of which in my experience of yoga students are Vata/Pitta and Pitta/Vata. Others include the Classic dual types –Vata/Kapha, Pitta/Kapha, Kapha/Vata, and Kapha/Pitta.

Ideally, each person needs to be able to receive and integrate the qualities of each dosha. By adjusting the yoga program, diet, and lifestyle according to current changes in one's life, one can minimize the "decaying" quality inherent in the doshas. Ayurveda seeks to maintain health and quickly regain it when it is lost. Yoga can supplement this goal, yet it is important to keep in mind that Classical Yoga's primary goal is spiritual transformation, not health. These two considerations need to be balanced or optimal adaptability is difficult to achieve.For our purposes, we will assume that we all possess qualities of each dosha, regardless of our predominant constitution, and that these qualities are expressed through our physical and psychological makeup.

Qualities of the Dual Constitutions

Vata/Pitta - This constitution tends to love yoga. I have observed that most students of yoga have this constitution or Pitta/Vata. They have an enjoyment of their body and naturally take to exercise to maintain their vitality. They become easily committed or attached to the practice depending upon their state of balance.

Vata/Kapha - This constitution tends to be quite healthy but is plagued with minor upsets that can create emotional havoc in their lives. It is an unsettling constitution in that one is constantly struggling to balance the extremes of their subtle and gross natures and desires.

Pitta/Kapha - This constitution is a lover of the senses and tends to be both healthy and robust.

Pitta/Vata –This constitution possesses the highest intelligence. Evolved PV can manifest change in their bodies when they fully understand their imbalance. The Vata quality can be ruled by the Pitta so changes can be experienced as transient.

Kapha/Vata –This large bodied person will have the most difficulty in maintaining their balance. They often have difficulties in facing their changeable emotional and mental states and in accepting things when they don't get their way. At the other extreme, they may be the kindest and most loving people we have had the pleasure of knowing.

Kapha/Pitta – This constitution, in addition to being charismatic, is the healthiest of all. Two illustrious yoga teachers, Prof. T. Krishnamacharya and his pupil Indra Devi, had this constitution and both lived to be over 100. Indra Devi passed away 3 weeks prior to her 103rd birthday. Both were wonderfully inspirational teachers for many people. For them, Yoga fine-tuned the natural gift of health with which they were blessed.

Those with an especially well-developed Pitta are blessed with the ability to easily transform. One client, a 23-year-old university student came to receive help with lower back pain. An Ayurvedic assessment found her to be Pitta/Vata constitution. I analyzed her discomfort as a unilaterally downward-rotated sacroiliac joint. I explained that she needed to rotate her right ilium forward so that when she lifted her leg in hip flexion, the sacroiliac joint would raise. I showed her a detailed anatomy book of this structure to clarify how the proper motion of the joint would occur and what muscles needed to be in harmony for its proper function. Upon presenting her with this new material, I saw her eyes flutter for a moment. This is the sign of a slower alpha brain wave pattern, normally associated with REM sleep or entering into a meditative state. My intuition told me that she had energetically adjusted herself. So I retested her and indeed her sacroiliac was moving properly without having to give her my "magic bullet" exercise to bring symmetry to this joint. [16]

Excess of Doshas

Diseases can be seen as an imbalance of the doshas in one of three forms: excess, diminished, or displaced (out of its home site). This fundamental view can help us to understand the basic properties of the elements comprising the doshas. Among the possible symptoms of excess are the following:

Vata	Pitta	Kapha
desire for heat	desire for cold	coldness
loss of memory	burning sensations	anemia
loss of adequate sleep	reduced sleep	excess of sleep
debility	fatigue	lethargy
dullness of the senses	bitter taste in mouth	excess salivation
skeletal pain	heartburn	pain in the chest
constipation	thirst	weight gain
blue skin	fair or yellowish skin	white coloration
increased peristalsis	inflammation	swelling
fainting	fever	heaviness
insensitivity to touch	poor vision	poor hearing
poor sense of smell	loss of sense of thirst	diminished sense of taste

Directing the Doshas toward Freedom

The doshas are constantly changing their effects upon the mind and body, and this change can be experienced as stress. Vata expresses itself as the element of change. It can create insight from its ability to clear away the fog of the denser doshas. When it is imbalanced, it produces fear. Fear of course is not always a bad emotion; for instance, when our survival is threatened fear helps to mobilize us to take action, protecting us from harm.

Pitta expresses itself as anger. We need to learn how to develop our own respiratory rhythm so that we can regulate our Vata and Pitta's naturally-protective qualities of fear and anger.

There is a famous story of the sadhu (a full time spiritual seeker) who lived in the forest in harmony with all the forces of nature and the animal kingdom, as well. He knew how to adapt to the cold of winter by variations of the heat-generating pranayama through the method of Bhastrika and to the hot of summer's intensity by the cooling pranayama Sitali. He had become even-minded by Ujjaye pranayama that kept his Vata in harmony. Through his mastery of mantra he learned the secret language of all the beasts. One of his friends was a venomous snake, who had become the scourge of the village and brought about many illnesses to unsuspecting gatherers of the forest's bounty. The snake's natural camouflage had made him undetectable to the villagers who sought to pick beneficial leaves and fruits for medicine and food. As a result, he was often stepped on and in his anger, bit many trespassers in his domain.

The sadhu decided the snake needed to learn to be free from causing harm (ahimsa) so he taught him how to do Brahmari pranayama. Through this pranayama, he turned his bite into a hiss. This saved him much grief. Through his hissing, he learned how to warn people of his presence so they wouldn't step on him by mistake as they had in the past.

The elevating quality of Kapha is stability and joyous harmony. Like the other doshas, it also has an imbalance, which causes decay and illness; yet, in proper proportion, it creates beneficial qualities. Kapha's core issue is closed-mindedness and attachment. When in harmony, this energy of attachment expresses itself as persistence, commitment, and love. In excess, it expresses as greed and self-centeredness; in deficiency, it is the inability to have stable relationships with others or ourselves.

Many of our difficulties in life arise from the wrong use of the mind. The challenge is to correctly utilize the tools our body and mind afford us in realizing the true nature of our Self.

The expression of Vata out of balance is ignorance. This ignorance is rooted in not knowing who we are. The resultant expression of that ignorance is having foolish, self-centered thoughts. In order to balance Vata, there must be a feeling of safety. Without this, there can be no openness to change. In each individual, this safety is found through insight into the labyrinth of interpretations their mind has given to life experiences.

With Pitta, the challenge is to avoid neglect of righteous duties. Harmonic Pitta gives us the vitality to perform our duties and all actions in a beneficial way, free from taking on the roles of others. One thus performs the tasks that are God-given.

For our Kapha attributes, the mind seeks to avoid misdirected endeavors that cause waste of energy, time, and resources. When in harmony, Kapha generates a stable, consistent lifestyle with faith in God's ever-present guidance. When imbalanced, the earth quality creates rigid thinking and attachment to possessions out of insecurity from only knowing a physical life.

Taken to extreme, these misguided forces will create harm to others and ourselves. In the <u>Yoga Sutras</u>, chapter two, the thirty-fourth sutra defines the qualities of harm and shows how they are deeply rooted in our psyche.

II, 34
Negative thoughts and emotions
are violent
in that they cause injury
to yourself and others
regardless of whether
they are performed
by you,
done by others,
or you permit them to be done.
They arise from greed,
anger, or delusion
and are indulged in
with either mild,
moderate, or excessive
emotional intensity.
They result in
endless misery and ignorance,
therefore by constantly cultivating
the opposite thoughts and emotions
the unwholesome tendencies
are gradually destroyed.[17]

The second sentence of this sutra refers to the dosha qualities. Greed is imbalanced Kapha, anger is imbalanced Pitta and delusion is imbalanced Vata. The recommended therapy cited in the subsequent sutras is cultivating positive attributes through affirmations and keeping good company. Each of the doshas has mental and emotional qualities that range from mildly stressful, to major eruptions in response to perceived threats and traumas. This stress is physiologically measurable whether the threats and traumas are real or imagined. Studies have shown that illness results from chronic perceptions of threat and the resultant overuse of the defense mechanisms of protection. The adage is that we can either fight, flight or freeze in response to stress. Fighting is a Pitta response, flight is a Vata response and freezing is a Kapha response.

Balanced Attributes of the Doshas

Negative (Imbalanced) Attributes of the Doshas

Vata	Pitta	Kapha
Fear	Anger	Attachment
Confusion	Overly-vocal	Incommunicative
Ignorance	Neglect	Seeks authority figures
Spaciness	Criticism	Misdirected endeavors
Anxiety	Judgment	
Panic attack	Rage/Violence	

Positive (Balanced) Attributes of the Doshas

Vata	Pitta	Kapha
Clarity	Energy	Nurturing
Intuition	Discrimination	Well - organized
Creativity	Enthusiasm	Committed
Quickness	Vitality	Trustworthy
Ability to adapt	Ability to digest	Ability to revere

The Three Doshas

Dosha	Effect of Balance	Signs of Imbalance	Aggravating Factors
Vata	Exhilaration Mind clear and alert Rhythmic functioning of bowels and menstrual cycle Proper formation of all bodily tissues Sound sleep Vitality	Rough skin Weight change Anxiety Worry Constipation Joint instability Arthritis Hypertension	Overwork Accidents Suppression of urges Winter season Emotional Suppression or over expression Fasting Pungent, astringent and bitter tastes
Pitta	Lustrous complexion Contentment Perfect digestion Softness of body Digestive mechanisms Balanced Brilliant intellect	Yellowish complexion Excessive body heat Insufficient sleep Heartburn Weak digestion Peptic ulcer Critical	Anger Strong sunshine Summer season Burning sensations Fasting Pungent, sour, or salty foods

Kapha	Stamina	Pale complexion	Daytime sleeping
	Normal joints	Coldness	Heavy foods
	Stability of mind	Excessive weight	Lack of exercise
	Dignity	Excessive sleep	Sugar
	Affectionate and	Dullness	Spring & Fall
	forgiving nature	Stiff joints	Sweet, sour, or salty
	Courage	Constipation	foods
	Regular exercise	Laziness	Greed or lust

Signs Vata is imbalanced

Vata-imbalanced individuals experience fatigue, loneliness, depression, and pain - especially dull chronic or irregular pains in the morning that leave after movement. One has the attitude that they can do things any way they like and "go with the flow."

How to balance Vata with Yoga

Emphasize asana that is done slowly, deliberately, and with great concentration. Extend the joints, make space and use an extremely soft, muscular effort. Specific vinyasas, which are done rhythmically at a slow breath pace with more emphasis upon breath than asana. Accentuate cool, soft Ujjaye pranayama, long and slightly audible.

Signs Vata is balanced

Feeling refreshed and relaxed. Breath is subtle yet moving deeply and fully into the lower abdomen. Colon is regular. There is an absence of pain. The mind is peaceful and enters meditation spontaneously, developing intuitive insights and understanding of others and self. One feels safe enough to know others intimately.

Signs Pitta is imbalanced

Pitta-imbalanced individuals have the attitude that things must be done the right way, often meaning their way. They criticize the way things happen to them or how others do things. There may be sudden bursts of anger or yelling to set right the wrongs of others. Conditions of inflammation arise in the skin, stomach, or eyes.

How to balance Pitta with Yoga

The practice of a creative sequence of asanas that stimulates them enough to feel alert yet not so stimulated as to become hot. Mild perspiration is good. One should feel the stretch in asana practice, but not the burn. In this way, they feel warmed, not over stimulated. Pranayamas like Bhastrika are beneficial when caution is heeded about keeping the heat confined to the Agni region of the middle abdomen.

Signs Pitta is balanced

Discrimination is developed between what is for the best and what they desire. The mind develops consideration for all aspects of life. One wants to serve others and gives freely in volunteer projects that elevate the community.

Signs Kapha is imbalanced

The Kapha-imbalanced individual has the attitude that things must be done "MY way." The body becomes large from excessive eating and lack of exercise and they begin to feel unhealthy. They experience laziness, lethargy, and lack of motivation to complete projects that have been underway for some time. Blood pressure will tend to rise and all physical activities will diminish. Lovemaking is seldom and one loses their capacity for pleasure.

How to balance Kapha with Yoga

Asana practice should be done for two purposes: to strengthen their body which generates stamina and to purify their physical tissues. Postures should be held long enough to challenge, but not so long as to strain. When done well, there is a feeling of vitality and joy returning to the practitioner. Devotional practices that open their heart and generate love are the best.

Signs Kapha is balanced

Their body is the picture of radiant health and nothing stops them from moving forward to accomplish their goals. Their commitment to a personal practice and personal relationships becomes more secure. There is self-confidence. Humility and devotion are signs of Kapha's evolution.

Tridoshic Balance and Imbalance

For Yogis, balancing the doshas is a lesser concern; their objective is to promote balance (sattva guna) so that the spiritual practices (sadhana) of the individual are deepened as the means to self-liberation (moksha). This takes the form of seeking to elevate the doshas into their evolutionary manifestations as prana, tejas, and ojas.

Imbalance of the doshas is a sign of lack of health, vitality, and enjoyment. Specifically, it manifests as a flow from one dosha to the next. Imbalance in Vata creates misunderstanding and misinterprets the situation, then moves to Pitta that criticizes and judges, then moves to Kapha to attach their own point of view and increase the strength of the ego.

What is tridoshic balance?

When all three qualities are most balanced, the result is optimal health on many dimensions.

Vata – Relaxation of the body
Pitta – Fire in the belly
Kapha – Warm, loving heart

III. The Classical Yoga Path

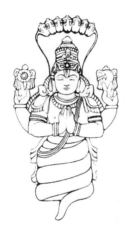

Overview of the Ashtanga

Where are you going?

In the course of life we sometimes move ahead blindly without thinking. As the commuting driver aggressively pushes ahead of his neighbor only to find the traffic light 100 feet ahead to be red. Where are we going in such a hurry, filled with rage when our short-sided objectives are obstructed? Rushing headlong filled with such short-sided objectives only to find our path obstructed. The pursuit of pleasure and the avoidance of pain are the simple answer. We seek to fulfill those desires that have been latently lingering incomplete. For otherwise we would be filled with frustration and anger.

For the Yogi the areas of life's destiny are fourfold: righteous action, wealth, sensual pleasures, and liberation. The practices of Classical Yoga can strengthen the body, restore health, purify the mind to an appropriate fulfillment of latent desires, and move the soul towards its ultimate communion with Spirit. The promises of Yoga are tremendous. These practices are among the most expedient ways to realize the potentials of life. Therealms in which we seek fulfillment are common to humanity. They are spoken of in many Vedic texts including the Guru Gita.

> *"I engage in the repetition of the Guru Gita*
> *to realize all the four values of life*
> *(dharma - righteousness; artha - wealth;*
> *kama - sensual pleasure; and moksha - liberation)."*[18]

Yoga holds the unique position in that it is the only Classical Indian philosophy that incorporates specific practices that have been proven over a lengthy history to purify the multi-dimensions of mind/body to leading an ethical lifestyle that is based on spiritual principles. It is indeed the practical aspect of the Vedic teachings. For through Yoga practices the philosophical ideals are utilized as the methods for the development of expanded awareness for a more fulfilling life.

There are innumerable ways in which the word Yoga can be understood. For the purpose of this book I shall be focusing upon definitions from the principal text of Classical Yoga, the Yoga Sutras of Patanjali. In the Krishnamacharya tradition, the arrangement of Patanjali's text into four chapters reveals "a personalized teaching for his four principal students. From this perspective, each chapter can be seen as an adaptation for a unique individual perspective. These can be seen as the archetypes of yoga students." [19]

Chapter One is especially for those students who have a predisposition for meditation as samadhi, hence the title Samadhi Pada (On Being Absorbed in Spirit). Chapter two is for Yoga students, who see that they have work to do on themselves. This chapter is entitled Sadhana Pada (On Practices for Being Prepared for Spirit). Chapter three, Vibhuti Pada (On Supernatural Abilities and Gifts), is for those students who seek to know the full potential of the mind. Chapter four,

Kaivalya Pada (On Absolute Freedom) is for the Yoga student who seeks only self-realization. For more details see my rendering of the <u>Yoga Sutras of Patanjali,</u> published by Weiser.

Chapter two's teachings are appropriate for 90% of Yoga students. Those students whose practice consists primarily of Yoga postures (asanas). This is the only chapter that describes these practices. For these students, the primary interest is the body, health, and freedom from physical suffering. This chapter is sometimes subtitled Kriya Yoga as this is given in the text of the first sutra of this chapter.

II, 1

The practical means
for preparing the desired state
of higher consciousness
consists of three components:
self-discipline and purification,
self study,
and living your life
as service
to the Lord. [20]

These three components, later defined as the final aspects of the ethical precepts (niyamas), are crucial; according to Krishnamacharya they form the foundation of Ayurvedic Yoga Therapy. For each of his archetypal students, Patanjali intends that they surpass their initial interest and manifest the full spectrum of their latent talents. In no other chapter is this more blatantly clear than in here, for the title comes across as an inducement to reach for Spirit. This chapter contains the famous eightfold path, a step by step guide from the outward-directed consciousness of the first five steps towards the inner-directed consciousness described more fully in chapter three.

Patanjali defines guideposts to keep the student of yoga progressing along the path. While there are numerous paths to Yoga, they have a common thread that has been delineated in the <u>Yoga Sutras</u>. In fact, the Sutras can be taken as a guide for anyone undergoing a discipline of body, breath, emotions, mind and spirit regardless of its cultural influence. Anyone proceeding any distance along this path cannot help but experience more joy and health. This state of fulfillment is what the yoga practitioner seeks to gain more consistently, more permanently.

Patanjali's Ashtanga Yoga, the tree of yoga has "eight limbs," and as he saw it, without any one, it would be a wounded tree.

II, 28

By sustained practice
of all the component parts of yoga,
the impurities dwindle away
and wisdom's radiant light
shines forth
with discriminative knowledge.

The eight component limbs of the Tree of Yoga are described in his <u>Yoga Sutras</u>
   II, 29 – III, 3: [21]
1) Yama – behavioral guidelines for conduct within society
   a. Non-violence (ahimsa): when mastered, one creates an atmosphere in
      which violence ceases.
   b. Truthfulness (satya): when perfected, one's words and deeds exist in ser-
      vice to that Truth.
   c. Abstaining from stealing (asteya): when mastered, that which is precious is
      drawn to you.
   d. Behavior that moves one towards the Truth (brahmacharya): when per-
      fected, then vitality is gained.
   e. Non-coveting (aparigraha): when mastered, knowledge of the hidden les-
      sons of the repetitive cycle of birth and death is gained.
2) Niyama - attitudes for personal discipline
   a. Purity (saucha): when established, there is a desire to protect your body
      and acessation of adverse contact with others.
   b. Contentment (santosha): when perfected, one gains supreme happiness.
   c. Perseverance in selfless service (tapas): when mastered, leads to a dwin-
      dling of all impurities and a perfection of the body, mind and sense or-
      gans.
   d. Study of the Self (svadhyaya): when mastered, leads to communion with
      your personal chosen ideals or deity.
   e. Devotion to God (Isvara pranidhana): when mastered, leads to absorption
      into the Divine Presence.
3) Asana - yoga posture
   When regularly practiced all movements end in a "steady and comfortable"
   pose, which is performed by relaxation of effort, and results in no longer being disturbed by duality's pulls – to reach for praise and avoid blame or many
   other polarities.
4) Pranayama - regulation of the in and outflow of breath/prana
   When perfected, one feels the life force (prana) permeating everywhere, transcending the attention given to either external or internal objects.
5) Pratyahara - withdrawal of the senses from their objects.
   When the senses become detached from external objects of the mind's desire

then the mind sees its source as pure consciousness.
6) Dharana - contemplation of one's true nature
   When mastered, the mind is confined to one place of attention.
7) Dhyana - meditation
   When mastered, a continuous flow of awareness to a single point of attention is maintained.
8) Samadhi - absorption in the Self

When achieved, it is the meditation that results in only the essential light of the object remaining; the object will have lost of its concrete form. The Spiritual Light prevails and is experienced as the essence of all of creation.

The first five steps are known as the outer path (bahiranga) and the final three the inner path (antaranga) in Yoga Sutras III, 7-8. Details of the inner path are not given for the chapter two student but reserved for the student whose spiritual practices are prescribed in chapter three.

The process of working on improving our selves through Yoga's various methodologies is known as sadhana. Sadhana for Tirumalai Krishnamacharya is the "means by which we obtain the previously unobtainable." [22]

The Three Paths of Yoga

The meaning of Yoga is to combine, unite, coordinate, or harmonize. The word "yoga" is derived from the word "yuj" which means either to unite or to separate: to unite with the real and separate from the unreal. The consonant "j" means "energy." The ultimate goal of yoga is to experience oneness or communion with the eternal energy.

There are three traditional Yoga paths: Jnana, Bhakti, and Karma.
   Head – Jnana Yoga   Heart – Bhakti Yoga   Gut – Karma Yoga

These three paths represent the most vital areas of life. We can see this perspective through the eyes of Ayurveda's energetic perspective of our psyche – head is Vata, heart is Kapha, and gut is Pitta.[23] The head is the path of intellect, seeking and finding Spirit as wisdom, Truth, timeless teachings. The heart is the path of devotion and higher emotions in which Spirit is expressed as love, faith, perseverance, and a connection to a greater sense of Self. The gut is the path of service as Spirit is found through acts of selfless service and doing one's duty for the benefit of humanity. In all cases the path is rooting out the core experience of the human being that of identify with the body.

According to the great sage Ramana Maharshi, ego is due to one possessing identification with their body.[24] Upon letting go of this false sense of self, a feeling of selflessness can arise and with it the nature of the True Self shines forth. This produces individual expressions of the Spiritual path in harmony with the individual's predispositions. When these are motivated by Vata then awareness of intellect and mind predominate. When motivated by Pitta then expressions of vitality and action are present. When Kapha is active then we are focused upon emotional aspects of being.

Another aspect of this is to examine the concept of the 5 bodies or vital sheaths (koshas) as delineated in the Taittiriya Upanishad II, 7. The densest body, annamayakosha is composed of food and is Kapha in nature. When awareness clings here we are drawn to look at our physical sensations and decide whether some form of physical activity is required. The second body, pranamayakosha, composed of prana is Vata in nature. Here our motivation is centered on needs for vitality and emotional health. The third body, manomayakosha, is also Vata in nature, though more subtle; we disregard bodily and emotional input and focus upon the content of our thoughts. If healthy we consider the health of our thoughts and the need for meditation and uplifting input. The fourth body, vijnanamayakosha, is Pitta in nature, manifesting as a spiritual light. Here discrimination has sorted out the vagaries of the mind; we are in a place of wisdom, seeking and finding timeless teachings. The fifth body, anandamayakosha, is the subtlest sense of ego as self. Here one transcends ordinary awareness yet still possesses a personal identity with the activities of the higher emotions of bliss and joy. While they are commonly experienced in hindsight as transcendent, not of one's own creation, these experiences in the moment are characterized with the sense of "I attained this bliss." It is only when the individual passes beyond these five bodies that the True Self is selfless, free of any agenda about body, energy, mind or emotions. Some teachers of meditation also acknowledge a sixth kosha, the asmitamayakosha, or the sense of "I."

Practices done from the first kosha generate sustaining health and well being. Those practices of the second kosha generate feelings of vitality and healing. The practices of the third kosha create positive attitudes, elevated self esteem and peace of mind. Those done in the fourth kosha result in intuitive insights, wisdom, and a direct perception of the truth of timeless teachings. The fifth kosha generates unique experiences of joy unrelated to any cause and effect. The sixth kosha generates a feeling of being pure consciousness without any form.

Kosha	Experience	Yoga Practices
Annamaya	Well being	Asana, satkarma Kriyas,
Pranamaya	Healing, emotional health	Sattvic diet, Ayurveda
Manomaya	Peace of mind	Restorative poses, pranayama,
Vijnanamaya	Wisdom, intuition	Sense withdrawal (pratyahara)
Anandamaya	Spontaneous joy	Ethical lifestyle (yama, niyamas)
Asmitamaya	Pure being (I-ness)	Meditation (dhyana), study of Self
Beyond the koshas	Transcendent True Self	Realization (svadhyaya)
		Spiritual absorption (samadhi)
		Witness consciousness
		Within all states of being

Yoga practices will purify the veiling aspect of each kosha. By maintaining a commitment to a multidimensional practice, the doshas become purified on each of these levels. However, it is possible to do a practice and not be grounded in the kosha related to its practice. For instance when we do yogasanas, we can focus on our physical body sensations and not gain full benefits. By maintaining a focus of feeling the stretch, strength may be diminished as I pointed out in Structural Yoga Therapy, Chapter 16. Similarly we can mentally direct our attention to the breath and its subtler component of prana, and by so doing enter the pranamaya-kosha and not reap the physical benefits we would have if our attention were upon strengthening a specific muscle. Instead we will be benefiting the vitality based energy body.

This points out the challenge the Yogini has in conveying Yoga Therapy, for her pathological and psychological conditions may be translated as symptoms of the corresponding kosha. Yet her perspective is that the symptoms might have their roots in a different dimension than has been diagnosed according to a different anatomical perspective. Some physical conditions have their roots in a subtler ko-sha and thus will not be touched by physical treatments whether they be traditional western medicine, Ayurvedic, or Yoga asana. If the physical disease's roots are in the unique ways their mind processes an experience, then meditation and/or psychotherapy is most beneficial. If the difficulty is held in the pranamaya sheath, no amount of asana or medicine or psychotherapy will remove its symptoms fully. This is true regardless of the medical or psychological diagnosis. If the challenge is due to a long standing karmic pattern, then only uncovering the karma and being willing to live life differently will change the situation.

The Yogini cannot therefore prescribe practices for western diagnoses because they are not cross correlated to her yogic anatomical perspective. And the opposite is also true, for the Yogini's diagnosis may not make sense to the western practitioner unless they are trained in the multidimensional perspective of Yoga anatomy.

I am often asked by phone or email to make yogic recommendations for specific conditions. I would love for this to be possible with accuracy. However, whether they are asking about physical conditions like herniated disc, mental like obsessive compulsive disorder (OCD), or loss of vital energy like chronic fatigue syndrome I cannot fully trust the diagnosis to be accurate within this scope. Therefore I need to see the individual, talk to them about their perception of their difficulty, feel their energy field, read their pulse, and then I can make accurate recommendations according to the unique constellation of symptomotology that person presents.

Each of the koshas can be seen as a defense mechanism that hides the True Self. We are all born with a common physiology and psychology but the miracle of God's creativity is that we are absolutely unique. The manifestation of this lack of connection with spirituality and our True Self is the identification we have with our body and its instability. The instability is natural, in Ayurvedic language it is called the doshas, literally "that which is unstable." These seeds of instability sprout to manifest presence of fear, anger, and attachment as the imbalance of each of the doshas. According to Yoga philosophy in its attempts to explain our challenge, this instability arises out of a primal motivator called the gunas (sattva - balance, rajas - activity, and tamas - inactivity).

Based on this perspective, the appropriate manner for removing the specific veils as defense mechanisms is this trilogy of Yogas.

Major Yoga Paths (Jnana, Karma, Bhakti) based on the Doshas

Jnana Yoga

Jnana (knowledge) Yoga is the way to self realization through spiritual knowledge. This is not the knowledge of material sciences or factual information but experiential knowledge gained by "knowing" the Self (atma vijnana). To achieve this knowledge we must silence the mind and go beyond its children, thoughts. Although this practice begins with thinking and meditation, the ultimate aim is to "silence the thought patterns of the mind" as detailed in the first chapter of Patanjali's Yoga Sutras.

The path of Jnana Yoga is expressed in several texts notably Yoga Sutras of Patanjali and the texts of Kashmir Shaivism. [25] The writings of Raja Yoga or the yoga of kings, as expounded in the Yoga Sutras is the directing of the mind toward Spirit. The first chapter of the Yoga Sutras contains the essence of Jnana Yoga. Raja Yoga is subdivided in the second chapter to preliminary practices using psychophysical techniques that can elevate the student towards the more complete path of Jnana Yoga. The preliminaries tersely described in the Yoga Sutras are Kriya Yoga, Ashtanga Yoga and Hatha Yoga.

Kriya Yoga as described in the opening sutra of the second chapter of the Yoga Sutras of Patanjali consists of three parts: energizing the will (tapas); self-study (svadhyaya); and surrender to God (Isvara pranidhana). Kriya means purification technique.

Ashtanga Yoga's "eight limbs" was described previously. Hatha Yoga can be seen as a subdivision of Ashtanga Yoga. It consists of physical postures and breathing techniques, the third and fourth limb of Ashtanga yoga. It is the school most westerners consider as yoga. The term "hatha" is composed of "ha" meaning the solar principle or sun and "tha" meaning the lunar principle or the moon. In the body, on the right side corresponds to the sun as an outgoing quality is dominant and on the left side corresponds to the moon as a receptive quality is dominant. Balancing these two principles by practicing asanas and pranayama, one can achieve this equilibrium and maintain lifelong health.

In the west Hatha Yoga is marketed under many names such as Power Yoga, Iyengar Yoga, Bikram Yoga, Sivananda Yoga, Integral Yoga, Jivamukti Yoga, Ashtanga Yoga of Pattabhi Jois, or Kripalu Yoga. Rarely is it called by its more traditional name of Hatha Yoga. For the beginner, there is often confusion as to the many different names of schools and styles of Hatha Yoga. Some practices are based on yoga teacher's names while others are based on the methods emphasized. In practice, the teaching of various Hatha Yoga schools differ in their approach to asana by coordinating breath with movement, aerobic ability, strength requirements, and stamina for the application of yoga postures. Most of these schools emphasize only the third limb, asana, of the outer practices of the eight limbs of Classical Ashtanga Yoga. Of notable exception to this are Sivananda Yoga, Integral Yoga, Jivamukti Yoga, and Kripalu Yoga where the "inner limbs," practices of meditation are a part of the standard curriculum.

Bhakti Yoga

Bhakti Yoga is the yoga of devotion. The aim of this yoga is to direct to the Divine love that lies at the base of every human heart. Devotion is expressed through the worship of the divine through rituals, chanting, and meditation.

The path of Bhakti Yoga is defined by Narada's Bhakti Sutras. Two editions are currently available – Narada Bhakti Sutras, Swami Tyagisananda, Madras: Sri Ramakrishna Math, 1967 and Narada's Way of Divine Love, Swami Prabhavananda, Hollywood: Vedanta Press, 1971. The path of Divine Love may include the energetic-based Tantra Yoga. Along these lines is The Path of the Mystic Lover by Bhaskar Bhattacharyaya with Nik Douglas and Penny Slinger, Rochester, VT: Destiny Books, 1993. In the Bible this path of love and faith are seen in the book of Job, which is a clear example of the fire of yogic tapasya, and the book following it the Psalms, an example of the other side of the Divine test. I would also recommend the writings of Swami Ram Das of Ananda Ashram in South India, Ammachi, and Abbott George Burke of Light of Christ Monastery, Borrego Springs, CA.

A more recent discovery of an exquisite example of Bhakti Yoga is the text the

Devi Gita. This fifteenth century text describes the Goddess as the primal being, the cause of creation, and describes the devotional means to attaining the experience of Her. The translator describes this text as a "work to supplant the famous teachings of Krishna in the Bhagavad Gita (the "Song of the Lord") from a Goddess inspired perspective." [26]

There are many different styles of Sanskrit that have been utilized over its 5000-year history. The particular style Patanjali uses in the Yoga Sutras is called by Vedic scholar David Frawley, the language of a lover of God (Bhakti). I see this especially in the first chapter's sutras on the Divine that are found in aphorisms 21-28. Patanjali implies that the science of union with the truth of your own Self must be approached reverently to uncover a pre-existing state of mind that is present behind thoughts and present regardless of one's constantly changing emotional or mental state.

Karma Yoga

Karma Yoga is yoga of selfless service. We can be doing this through humanitarian efforts such as helping to uplift the needy and to work for humanity. Mother Theresa, Mahatma Gandhi, Martin Luther King, and Florence Nightingale are fine examples of those who practiced this yoga in their lives.

The path of Karma Yoga is most clearly expressed in the Bhagavad Gita. Of the numerous editions available, my favorites are these four – The Song Celestial – 42 verses selected as the principle teachings and reset by Ramana Maharshi, Ramana Ashram, 1995; The Gita According to Gandhi – Anasaktiyoga by Mohandas K. Gandhi, San Francisco: Dry Bones Press, 1993; Bhagavad-Gita - Thus Sang Lord Krishna by Sant Keshavadas, Tyler, Texas: All Faith Fellowship, 1975; God Talks with Arjuna – the Bhagavad Gita by Paramahansa Yogananda. Los Angeles: Self Realization Fellowship, 1995. Other prominent writings on this path are Karma Yoga by Swami Vivekananda.

Apex of the Doshas equated to Yoga Sutras II, I

Prana, Tejas and Ojas

Through the process of balancing then evolving the doshas – Vata, Pitta, and Kapha – their subtle elements become generated. These are respectively called Prana, Tejas and Ojas. Vata, Pitta, and Kapha relate to the gross functions of breath, digestion, and physical health. The subtler essence relates to the soul's desire for Spirit, higher intelligence, and devotion to the Source. It is this transformation that the Ayurvedic practitioner seeks through her/his cultivation of the life science. For the Yogi these are naturally arising from doing elevated practices and being in the company of illuminated souls.

This form of Prana is different than those mentioned previously in the subdoshas. This Prana is the physical essence of Spirit as it manifests in the body. Prana evolves from the balance of the subtle functioning of the physiology and seeks to go beyond the identification of the self with the body. Prana imparts to the ordinary tissue and mind the ability to adapt to change, creativity, and imparts the desire for one's evolution. Prana provides us with the desire to procreate, the will to live and to sustain life. It is the breath of life imparted to the individual through live organic foods. It results in the feeling of connectedness to the cycle of life. In the mind it manifests as peace.

From a healthy Pitta dosha comes the fire of discernment that directs one toward the good and creates indifference to that which is destructive. This is known as tejas. This individual instinctively knows the difference between healthy and unhealthy activities and is able to make consistent choices to better themselves and those they serve. Tejas is the discriminative factor of the being that results from a spiritual illumination. It is the fire of higher intelligence that builds one's passions to know the truth of human existence. It is the one that asks, "Who am I? and why am I here?" It manifests as the spiritual quest and the craving for living in the light of Spirit.

Ojas builds upon the foundation of a balanced Kapha as physical and emotional strength and stamina into creating a vibrant, healthy immune system. This strength, stamina, and health leads to an open heart – it is much more than physical health and the absence of pain. Ojas manifests physically as our sexual fluids and additionally in women, it is the life giving force of a mother's good heart becoming breast milk. Its fullest expression is love of all life.

These three forces are more interrelated than the tridoshas. While it is true that an imbalanced Vata will lead to Pitta and Kapha derangements, an excess or diminishment of Prana, Tejas, or Ojas will more immediately change the others. Low ojas will tend to excite prana and tejas. While increased prana tends to dry out ojas, diminished prana tends to make ojas less able to flow.

IV. Yoga Lifestyle

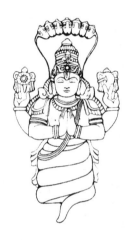

Yoga's spiritual practices (sadhana) form the foundation for the Yogi's lifestyle. As you deepen your practice, the concept of integrity becomes clearer and the Yoga student with integrity will find that the yamas and niyamas support their ethical actions at bearing good fruit. The practice of Yoga needs support from a lifestyle that is conducive to sustaining the subtle and sometimes not so subtle changes that good practice naturally creates. Among the areas of change you might need to consider are the following:

Daily Schedule

This aspect of lifestyle is the most important. Regularity promotes a natural capacity to balance Vata's underlying energy of prana thus stabilizing the mind and physiological rhythms. Optimal is to keep your same schedule regardless of external events that might be beyond your control, such as travel for work or holiday vacations. I find that when I travel, I maintain a healthy balance by immediately changing my watch to the new time zone as soon as I am on the plane. For the number of hours of zone difference, I meditate or do mantra repetition (japa) that many hours during the flight. I find that taking the time to do this balances me and it minimizes the stress of my current schedule of frequent air travel.

Having a set time for meals, sleep, exercise, meditation and prayer makes all the difference in the world for promoting unity consciousness. The world is the same no matter where we travel; around the block, outside the home, or to distant countries. There is no difference in people - only in climate. and for this we may need to make adjustments as one would adjust for the seasonal changes that have their rhythms.

Seasonal Changes

The opening verses of folk singer Pete Seeger's famous song come from Ecclesiastes III, 1-5 -

> *"To every thing there is a season, and a time to every purpose under heaven:*
> *A time to be born and a time to die: a time to plant and a time to sow:*
> *A time to kill and a time to heal: a time to break down, and a time to build:*
> *A time to weep, and a time to laugh; a time to mourn, and a time to dance:*
> *A time to cast away stones, and a time to gather stones together: a time to embrace, and a time to refrain from embracing."*

The rhythms of life have a need that they serve; to promote harmony and adaptability. When we adapt well we are reflecting a balance of Vata dosha. For the Yogi, the challenge of life's spontaneity reveals their capacity for dispassion to act according to the situation.

Diet

In the book, <u>The 3 Season Diet</u>,[27] Dr. John Douillard expertly lays out Ayurvedic guidelines in a practical manner to encourage adjusting diet to our region's seasonal rhythms. In the winter, a diet promoting diminishing Vata to balance its tendency to be dry and cold. In spring and fall, a diet for diminishing Kapha and its tendency to be cool and wet. In summer, a diet for diminishing Pitta and its tendency to become overly heated.

The desire for healthy, natural and organic food is to be encouraged. When the doshas are balanced, the natural result will be expressed in your appetite craving healthy foods. When the doshas are unstable, we make less ideal choices. Often these less ideal decisions are based on what we interpret our taste buds are craving. Nutritional education is an important aspect of lifestyle that engages some people their entire lives. Others understand the basic principles easily and can act quickly to restore harmony when adaptation is required. Still others are slow learners, continuing to make the same mistakes and suffer similar consequences to their digestive organs. Let us all learn efficiently and change our lifestyle to support dietary insights. Remember that the Sanskrit word for food, anna, means Mother, and we are all nurtured by Mother Earth. It is within our power to allow Her to nurture us with Her best produce.

Expression of Natural Urges

A healthy person is appropriately emotional. They feel sympathy for others without losing their sense of self. When someone dies they are sad; when a joyous occasion arises they are happy. Emotional expression is the juice of life.

In the same way that emotional health is maintained by its natural expression, so also the Yogi encourages biological urges to be free. As the classical Ayurvedic text, Caraka Samhita says, "One should not suppress the natural urges relating to urine, feces, semen, gas, vomiting, sneezing, belching, yawning, hunger, thirst, tears, sleep and breathing caused by over exertion. Various types of diseases occur by the suppression of these urges." [28] The <u>Caraka Samhita</u> goes onto explain various remedies for the problems that arise from the suppression of these urges.

Urges to be Suppressed

Both the <u>Yoga Sutras</u> and the <u>Caraka Samhita</u> mention negative actions (yamas) that are to be suppressed. One wants to naturally avoid causing harm and so those harmful acts should be suppressed whether they seek expression mentally, verbally or physically. "A wise person should refrain from satisfying the urges relating to greed, grief, fear, anger, vanity, shamelessness, jealousy, too much of attachment and malice. One should also refrain from letting loose the urges of speaking extremely harsh words, back-biting, lying and the use of untimely words. The virtuous one, who is free from all vices relating to mind, speech and physical actions, is indeed happy and he alone enjoys the fruits of virtue (dharma), wealth (artha) and desire (kama)." [29]

This practice cultivates the emotion of dispassion, cited by Patanjali (Yoga Sutras I, 12) as being the secret for the attainment of success in Yoga sadhana. The middle ground cultivated by this practice helps to establish the attitude conducive for spiritual insight and revelation. One can easily see how the Buddha became "the illuminated One" based on his years of Yogic discipline prior to finding his own path.

Relationships

Relationship is Yoga. Yoga is relationship. Both qualities in natural expression promote harmony. When harmony is present, so is Yoga. When Yoga is present, we will tend to be in right relationship with all aspects of life. I have seen in my private Yoga Therapy practice a high percentage of students suffering from lower back pain have preexisting conflicts in their intimate relations. Taking time out for healthy communication exercises with our business and intimate partners can go a long way to promoting a stress free life. Time out can remove the difficulties that naturally arise with not being understood or not clearly expressing your truth. Both sexes need their partner to express themselves in ways that show they are fulfilled or making progress toward their commonly held goals. Communication is a prime directive for a healthy relationship. And yet both sexes need different types of communication to fulfill their goal of sensual and sexual pleasure (kama).

Intimacy and Sexuality

A healthy relationship invites a happy sex life. Men who are sensitive lovers know that intimacy and deep communication are foreplay to a women's heart. When a woman is met eye to eye and heart to heart in intimate conversation, she is naturally aroused and will express her passion freely. Women who are good lovers know that when they express praise and pride in their mate's accomplishments, their lovers will feel the effects of more testosterone. When a man feels good about his projects and creativity, he is passionate and experiences love. Find out what expresses love to your partner. Rarely is it the same for both partners. By giving what your partner wants instead of what you want them to give you; you will experience selfless service and love.

No technique is needed for healthy love making. Partners need to understand the differences between making love and having sex. Both are important natural urges and yet lead to tremendously different benefits. Detrimental emotional and physical effects will arise if they are not expressed. Sharing physical love is a gift of human and divine Grace.

Celibacy

Celibacy is an appropriate condition for select periods of life - when one is away from home on a work assignment, during periods of depth study and reflection, when you or your partner is ill, or to promote self discipline for a specified period of time. In case of illness, sexual expression may be limited to hugs and words of affection. This period is appropriate for promoting the energies of healing. Or if sexual expression is desires in such times, it can be limited to gentle intercourse (increasing Kapha) with no stimulation of Pitta resulting in climax. This method of intercourse or continence is promoted in some yogic schools. They consider it the fourth vow of self control (the vow of brahmacharya as an aspect of yama) for both partners are retaining the life force for healing and/or spiritual elevation.

On-going Study

Life is an ever-evolving eternal cycle that reveals an inherent need to realize our potential. The more we understand that learning is never ending, the easier it is to know that Yoga is a lifelong practice that can tremendously benefit our evolution. A commitment to an uplifting lifestyle that enhances our capacity for sustained service to others makes life worth while. Yoginis and Yogis are those who life a lifestyle for their upliftment and for service to others. Another definition of a Yogini is one who is selfless.

Ethics for a Yogic Lifestyle

Patanjali, as the codifier of the tradition before him, realized the importance of ethics not only for maintaining a healthy society but also for the evolution of the individual. He saw the process of Yoga as one of coming to know yourself, out of which would naturally arise energy and enthusiasm which would re-vitalize society in its concern for welfare of the common good. This ancient system is known as the Sanatana Dharma, or the Eternal Path of Righteousness. Yogis know that life is a spectrum; all benefit from uplifting any single person.

The community represents the first level of this Higher Power. By thinking of others and how they are impacted, pettiness is removed and the mind is naturally lifted up. The burden of the sense of self and the depression of feeling isolated is lightened, with increased connection to Spirit. However, Patanjali knew that certain activities must be avoided or society would be destroyed.

Disciplines for self control (yamas)

Of the eight limbs of Classical Ashtanga Yoga, the first two means of sadhana are the attitudes that project the direction for one's lifestyle. With it they also determine one's capacity to remain in integrity with the challenges that life will naturally present.

They are for the purpose of restraining the ego so that it can appreciate an serve others. Conscious practice of the yamas restores all virtues.

Self control (yama) consists of five principles:
    non-violence,
    truthfulness,
    freedom from stealing,
    behavior that respects
    the Divine as omnipresent,
    and freedom from greed.[30]

The first concept of the first limb (the five yamas), nonviolence, is considered the prime directive. It can be equated to the Bible's golden rule "Do unto others as you would have them do unto you." This quality is the most important of all the attitudes for Yoga. It is nothing less than altruism - a selfless regard for the well being of others. When this factor is taken into consideration first all our actions will be beneficial to others and ourselves. Without this quality our actions will be self-centered. From self-centeredness will inevitably arise all sorts of dis-ease. From this erroneous approach, the mind and our biologically based chemistry change generating states of anxiety or depression due to its false interpretations of life situations. Health and dis-ease are the manifestation of the state of our mind.

The opposite of self-centeredness, altruism creates empathy, the capacity for feeling and responding to others as if they are our self. Mahatma Gandhi translated ahimsa not as nonviolence but as love; and this forms the basis of true spirituality. The intention necessary for Yoga is to live its teachings not merely perfect the practices.

The second principle of the yamas, truthfulness or satya, is built upon this foundation. "According to a recent study conducted by the University of Connecticut, the average American tells 26 lies every day." [31] I don't know who the "average American" is, but this study certainly points out a major moral deficiency. When one speaks the truth and lives with integrity, none of the signs of falsehood that generate physical, mental, and emotional stress exist. Among the subtle yet easily recognizable signs of lying mentioned in the study are taking "sworn oaths, peculiar body language, unverifiable facts, shifty eyes, verbal stumbling, and absurd claims." Where does it end? Yoginis seek to be good at knowing the truth and speaking and acting in accordance with that truth. This is not easily attained in a culture where the average person lies 26 times a day. Despite that, Yoga sadhana calls for speaking the truth and maintaining integrity. Together these two form the basis of Yoga lifestyle. The other eight principles of the Yoga code of ethics will naturally arise from one who is in integrity with these first two.

Observances (niyamas) for personal practice

Patanjali inherited the tradition of virtues that are to be cultivated for the upliftment of both the society and the individual. The five niyamas uplift the yogastudent to becoming an individual focused upon helping others. They are -

> purity,
> contentment,
> self-discipline and purification,
> Self study,
> and devotion to the Lord. [32]

These ten principles are the foundation for a spiritual life. Without constant vigilance to them, that which is attained towards the fulfillment of the four goals of life can be easily lost washed out to the seas of worldliness. It is not that worldliness is bad, simply that without leading a spiritual lifestyle, benefits arising from the external world are all short lived. Spiritual benefits are durable.

My spiritual preceptor, Swami Prakashananda, revealed in private conversation that it is possible for one to fall from the Grace of illumination. He said that no attainment is solid enough to be safe from harm. One should be vigilant, even after having regular, profound spiritual experiences that might be perceived as Self Realization. One can lose even the attainment of spiritual illumination, which he said is given by God's Grace. This is an affirmation of Krishnamacharya's rendering of Yoga Sutras I, 23 "The end of spiritual practice is only attained by placing oneself in the Lord." [33] Therefore, one should be constantly vigilant, not only for criticizing others but also watchful for your maintenance of the vows through an ethical lifestyle.

Through the consistency of these vows, the Yogini becomes transformed and the world appears as a blessed place wherever they go, whatever they do. Jnaneshwar Maharaj said, "He is a true human being who understands that this entire world is his home. His family is the family of God. Such a person has true wisdom." [34]

One of my favorite prayers is the Universal Prayer, composed from various Upanishads by my guru. Its opening stanza is as follows –

> *May all of the wicked return to good,*
> *May all who are good obtain true peace.*
> *May all who are peaceful be freed from bonds,*
> *May all who are free set others free.* [35]

This beautiful prayer describes the qualities of human evolution as attained by Yoga Sadhana. May our upliftment lead to the upliftment of all we encounter.

The essence of all the vows of Yoga is contained in the first precept of the yamas called ahimsa, non-violence. In Sudbury, a suburb of Boston, there is a wonderful shrine and contemplative grounds called the Peace Abbey (www.peaceabbey.org). The central figure of the shrine honoring the names of a hundred peacemakers is Mahatma Gandhi. When asked to define ahimsa, Gandhi translated it not as non-violence but as love. To be truly non-violent we must move beyond stopping our rage and insensitivity, to a positive expression of their opposite.

Ethics causes us to contemplate the significance of our actions. By self-observation and deliberation we strive to lead a life in humility to the Higher Power. Without Humility to a Higher Power, the mind is lost in the inevitable emotional soup of fear, anger, or attachment (the imbalances of Vata, Pitta, and Kapha) because it is dominated by a self-serving ego. Humility is the act of surrender to the authority and grace of the Higher Power.

According to the <u>Bhagavad Gita</u>

> *Brooding on sense objects*
> *causes attachment to them.*
> *Attachment breeds craving;*
> *craving thwarted causes anger.*
>
> *From anger is born delusion;*
> *delusion is the source of loss of memory of the Self.*
> *Loss of spiritual memory causes the decay of discrimination.*
> *From the decay of discrimination,*
> *annihilation of spiritual life follows.* [36]

A few chapters later the Gita gives us this remedy of the problem.

> *Verily, nothing in this world is as sanctifying as wisdom.*
> *In due course of time, the devotee who is successful in yoga*
> *will spontaneously realize this within his own Self.* [37]

V. Sattvic Yogic Diet

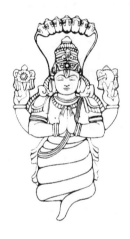

Of all the factors for physical health, none is as important as the formation of the tissues through the remarkable process called digestion. The ancient Vedic teachings called the physical body, the annamayakosha which literally means "that which is made of food." A common saying is that we are what we eat. The same is true even before we eat it. According to Vasistha's Yoga, IV: 15 page 155 "the jiva or living soul became the food that entered the body of the sage Bhrigu, and was later reborn as Sukra." In the Taittiriya Upanishad, the sage Bhrigu reveals, "food is God." He goes on to say that from food, life springs forth, by food it is sustained and in food, it merges when departed. Further, he says in 1.5.3 "indeed, all the vital forces are nourished by food."

Certainly, the quality of food that we ingest is very important. Though foods are made of chemical components, we must remember the Yogic and physicists point of view that matter and energy are interchangeable. The presence of life force (prana) in foods is crucial to the vitality of the multi-dimensional body/mind. To live better through advances in chemistry by taking primarily altered, "improved" food is extremely short-sighted thinking that ignores the omnipresence of the life force.

The medieval Yoga text, the Gheranda Samhita, a collection of writings by the sage Gheranda, states that "he who commences the practices of Yoga without first controlling his diet becomes a victim of many diseases. His Yoga does not succeed . . . Half of the stomach should be filled with food, the first quarter with water, and the fourth part should be left free for the movement of air." [38]

Krishna, in the Bhagavad Gita, makes more specific recommendations about diet. Here, he describes the benefits of eating a diet that is balancing to the sattva guna (principle of harmony) and cites the effects of foods that either increases rajas or tamas guna (principles of over stimulation or lethargy).

- Foods, in the mode of sattva, increase the duration of life, purify existence, give strength, and increase health, happiness, and satisfaction. Such foods are juicy and fatty. They are very conducive to the healthy condition of the body.
- Food that is too bitter, too sour, too salty, too pungent, too dry or too hot causes distress, misery, and disease. Such food is very dear to those in the mode of rajas.
- Foods prepared more than three hours before being eaten, which are tasteless, juiceless, and decomposed, which have a bad smell, and which consists of remnants and untouchable things are very dear to those in the mode of tamas.[39]

A sattvic diet is ideal for those who are practicing yoga on a daily basis. It should consist mainly of fresh fruits, vegetables, and grains. Aim to use little dairy (except from farms that truly love cows and will not traumatize them with the fear of life ending in slaughter) and wheat, as they tend to be allergens. There are some foods that are tridoshic, or beneficial to everyone, as they help restore balance to all the doshas. They are the least likely to offend allergy prone individuals. These foods are basmati rice either white or brown, ghee (freshly made at home from healthy happy cows), and buckwheat (kasha).

When nourishment is pure, sattva as the instrument of wisdom,
becomes pure and when sattva is purified,
then the power of meditation becomes stabilized. [40]

Whenever possible a Yogi's foods should be organically grown. The healthiest I have ever experienced myself to be was when I lived in the redwood forests of northern California and ate a diet of 90% organic food, locally grown. The coastal redwood forests are full of Prana and my diet was also saturated in this Prana. It wasn't long before I could literally experience my "city diet taste buds" falling off. My tongue regained its youthful red color, I had plenty of vitality, and I felt fantastic. My sensitivity to the force of life was at its peak.

For meals to be sattvic, they should be taken at a regular time. My recommendations are to have a breakfast that is moderate in size with plenty of fresh fruits. Lunch is the main meal with both increased quantity and heavier to digest food. This is the time when agni is at its peak, so your digestive fire is ready to do its work. The meal should consist of proteins from grains and legumes, fresh vegetables and light amounts of dairy or cheese.

Your environment can also greatly contribute to having a sattvic experience. Find ways to enjoy the food preparation, whether it is with music you enjoy or quiet time to listen to the sounds of nature. To a great extent, the health of your body is determined by the health of your mind. Whenever possible, I enjoy preparing my food and chanting the Hare Rama mantra I learned while living in ashrams. By projecting the vibratory energy of the mantra into the food and my belly I find I am more sensitive to what is truly better food and the love of my spiritual practice is transferred into the food.

The sound Ram is the seed source (bija mantra) for the third chakra. That is the home of the digestive fire, agni. Singing this chant has always brought my mood up and the Prana of my heart begins to enjoy the aroma of my food. This is the foretaste of delights yet to come. When I cannot eat at home, I do my best to eat in restaurants and/or homes where I am greeted with smiling faces. The love and friendliness of the servers and cooks is also part of the prequel to a happy, healthy diet. Friendship makes even pizzas tastefully plugged into their pranas.

When you are eating out, the atmosphere is beyond your control, but the internal atmosphere is always within your control. So take a few moments to sit quietly and do gentle wave breathing from head to abdomen (ujjaye pranayama). Focus upon your abdominal region during this period and wait until your belly has settled before making your decision about what to request for your meal. Waiters are a crucial component as much as the cook is in creating a harmonious environment for enjoyment and nutrition. My favorite restaurants are those where I know the waiters by name and we are involved in sharing life not merely a meal.

There should be plenty of fresh natural spring water in your diet. Ideal would be to live in an environment where the running spring water would be readily available. Second best is to get bottled water or distilled water. The ideal water will have a distinctively delicious sweet taste. Sweet tasting water has plenty of prana and promotes healing.

Fasting is not recommended for Yoga sadhana except in the case of illness. However, Kapha predominant people or those with Kapha diseases will receive the most benefit from experienced guidance on using purification diets and fasting. If you do fast then I caution you to be extraordinarily careful the second and third day following the fast. Be sensible and eat moderately at this time for your mind and emotions, not your physiology, will be expressing their hunger.

Dietary Precautions

Extra hot or spicy foods are rajasic. Foods that tend to produce excess gas (increasing Vata) like broccoli, large beans like kidney or lima, and undercooked cabbage are rajasic. The effects of foods can of course be changed by various methods of preparation and slowing down your ingestion rate if you have an increased Vata. Steaming vegetables or cooking beans with digestive spices such as ginger can eliminate the gaseous properties of these foods as well (making them easier to digest). These foods in general will aggravate Vata and Pitta. The purification practices described in this book are especially beneficial for those with digestive problems.

Foods that are prepackaged (canned or boxed); leftovers that have been stored for more than 24 hours in the refrigerator or have artificial preservatives are tamasic. When you need to add spices to food to suit your taste buds, suspect that it is tamasic.

To be on the safe side, always look for the feelings of prana, or vital life force, within your diet. Hold the food in your hands for a moment before dropping it in your shopping cart. If you cannot feel the life force, pass it by.

Vegetarian Diet

"In meditation, the inner energy first purifies your body. By eating meat, you are making the body impure again; so there is more work for the energy to do. If you want to reach higher stages of meditation quickly, it would be better to give up meat." [41]

While vegetarianism is not a requirement for yoga practice, a vegetarian diet improves your capacity to receive the most benefit from Yoga. It is the most healing diet as it is low in fat and free from cholesterol. "A vegetarian diet reduces obesity, constipation, lung cancer, alcoholism, increased high blood pressure of hypertension, coronary artery disease, diabetes type II, and gallstones. People on an animal protein diet are twice as likely to develop gallstones." [42] In general, food from the carcasses of animals is tamasic and will increase toxicity (ama). I am haunted by a quotation from Oliver Wendell Holmes, the former Supreme Court Justice. When asked why he was a vegetarian, he replied, "I do not want to make my body a graveyard for dead animals." A blunt statement of the obvious truth.

Not only is a vegetarian diet more beneficial for health, it also tends to promote a balance in the doshas which increases a sense of peace during meditation. My guru did not require a vegetarian diet, though it was all that was available in his meditation centers and residential communities.

Anti-Ama Diet

Focus on a plan that minimizes the toxicity of the body and allows it to become restored to feelings of youthful vitality. Ama is the waste products of incomplete digestion that will create tissue toxicity. The word literally means "not Mother" or "not nurturing." It arises from eating improper foods and/or eating at irregular hours, both of which contribute to a diminished digestive fire.

Ama has similar properties to Kapha dosha; therefore, an anti-Kapha diet of bitter and pungent foods will assist in detoxification of the tissue cells. This is best considered as a short term cleansing process. Sour fruits like grapefruit or lemons are particularly beneficial in the morning. For lunch the meal can be supplemented with vegetable juices made from celery, parsley, spinach, alfalfa and carrot. Grains, particularly couscous and buckwheat (kasha), are also cleansing. The evening meal can consist of soup and salad. The meals should be spiced strongly with cayenne, black pepper, ginger or bitter herbs. Herbs such as gentian or golden seal are helpful for removing ama.

The best long-term treatment for ama in the system is preventative; balancing your lifestyle through sustained regularity in sleep, exercise, meals, and work. When any of these is not under control, it's especially important to maintain the others. A balanced lifestyle generates harmonious Vata, disciplined self-effort generates harmonious Pitta, and regulated taste generates balance in Kapha.

Ayurvedic Responses to Taste

The tongue's taste buds are sensitive enough to distinguish 6 areas, each of which can detect a different taste sensation. There are six specific tastes that can be detected on the frontal region of the tongue: sweet, salty, sour, bitter, astringent, and pungent.[43] Only the first four tastes are recognized in Western physiology texts, though some researchers describe alkaline and metallic as additional tastes. [44]

Sweet receptors are most plentiful near the tip of the tongue. It is interesting to note that the taste threshold, the minimum amount of a substance necessary for recognizing a taste, is highest for sweet taste. They are the lowest in sensitivity, and require the most food for perceiving that sensation; thus it is easy to overeat sweet foods before you notice that you are sated. Salt is perceived immediately behind the tip of the tongue on both sides; sour taste is located just behind that region on both sides of the tongue, (though in some individuals, the sensors for salt and sour taste overlap); bitter is detected at the back of the tongue and is the highest in sensitivity. "The relative taste thresholds are 10 units for bitter, 100 for sour, 2000 for salt and 10000 for sucrose sugar." [45] "Each taste bud usually has a greater degree of sensitivity to one or two of the taste sensations than to the others . . . The bitter taste buds provide a protective function, for they detect principally the poisons in wild plants." [46]

My guru, Swami Muktananda, was a master chef who followed Ayurvedic principles in composing the ashram diet. He would often come into the ashram's kitchen and "polish" the cook's work. He explained that the ideal cooked food's taste should strike all the taste bud centers evenly, serving as a moderate uniform stimulation to the entire frontal surface of the tongue. He could play with small amounts of salt, lemon, and sugar to create a remarkable chemistry in the enormous pots of vegetables or grains in order to elicit this taste response.

In Ayurvedic cooking, therapeutic tastes are based on reducing the predominant dosha and creating sattvic balance. Three tastes increase each of the three doshas and three decrease them, according to the elements that they are made of. Vata is most increased by bitter taste, then astringent and pungent. It is decreased most strongly by salty taste, then sour and sweet.

Sour is the best taste for Vata.

Pitta is increased primarily by sour, then pungent and salty. It is most decreased by bitter taste, then astringent and sweet. Bitter is the best taste for Pitta.

Kapha is most increased by sweet taste, then salty and sour. It is diminished strongest by pungent taste, then bitter and astringent. Pungent is the best taste for Kapha.

Taste	Example	Effect
Sweet	Sugars, starches, wheat	Mild cooling, ↑ K, ↓ V P
Salty	Sea food, seaweed	Mild heating, ↑ K P, ↓ V
Sour	Acidic fruits, yogurt	Moderate heating, ↑ P K, ↓ V
Bitter	Dandelion, rhubarb	Strongly cooling, ↑ V, ↓ P K
Pungent	Hot spices, ginger, coffee	Strongly heating, ↑ P V, ↓ K
Astringent	Beans, lettuce, alfalfa	Moderately cooling, ↑ V, ↓ P K

Tastes and the Doshas

Sweet - Sweet taste is mildly cooling, strongly increases Kapha, mildly decreases Vata and Pitta. This taste is particularly good for children, seniors, and those who are recovering from injuries, as this form of increase to Kapha will tend to nourish and strengthen body tissues. This promotes healing as it improves the immune system. It is the foundation for ojas, a subtle energy that promotes health on all three dimensions - physical, emotional, and spiritual. Sweet taste can relieve thirst. We commonly see that as people age, the vitality of their senses diminishes. As a result, the sensation of thirst is often misperceived as a desire for something sweet to eat. Thus instead of promoting a balance in Kapha, the body tissue increases and lethargy is promoted by a misconstrued desire for sweet.

Sweet taste is predominant in sugars like cane and maple syrup (which are cooling), beet sugar and honey (both are heating), rice, milk, dates, licorice, and oils from seeds and nuts. It is most balanced in whole grain starches.

In excess, it can damage the spleen or pancreas and cause hypoglycemia or diabetes. It will contribute to excessive weight gain, lethargy, loss of appetite, cough, and insomnia. In general its over consumption promotes the aging process.

Salty - This taste is mildly heating, mildly increases Kapha, mildly increases Pitta, and strongly decreases Vata. It stimulates salivation and digestion and works as a sedative and in larger quantities is a laxative. It can alleviate stiffness in small quantities. It is naturally occurring in mineral salts and seafoods, shellfish and seaweeds.

When excessive, it can damage the kidneys and cause edema or hypertension. It can thus over stimulate Pitta causing weakness, wrinkles, hair loss, and inflammatory skin diseases. On the other side of the issue, cramping is a sign of a Vata imbalance often caused by a lack of sea salt or diminished mineral absorption.

Sour - This taste is moderately heating, strongly increases Pitta, mildly increases Kapha, and moderately decreases Vata. It increases appetite, digestion, thirst, elimination, and diminishes Vata to release gas. It is a beneficial taste for promoting sensory awareness and mental acuity. It is available in citrus fruits, berries, sour fruits like pineapple, cheese, hibiscus and rosehips tea, and fermented foods such as yogurt and kefir.

Too much sour taste causes acidity, burning sensation and bleeding; in the long run it can cause gastritis or peptic ulcers. It also increases sensitivity in the teeth, edema, ulcers, and heartburn.

Bitter - Bitter taste is strongly cooling, strongly increases Vata, strongly decreases Pitta, and moderately decreases Kapha. It can be cleansing to the taste buds as it causes a withdrawal reaction making them discharge excessive tastes that were over stimulated. It is a remedy for fainting, itching, reducing fevers and burning sensations. Bitter taste is found in herbs such as gentian root, dandelion root, fenugreek, and goldenseal as well as rhubarb.

Bitter taste taken excessively causes coldness in hands and feet, vertigo, emaciation; continued excessive use may damage the heart to cause anemia, low blood pressure or insomnia.

Pungent – This taste is strongly heating, moderately increases Pitta, mildly increases Vata, and strongly decreases Kapha. Because it increases Pitta, it can improve mental acuity, appetite and digestion as well as improving the taste of food. It helps eliminate excessive Kapha and is helpful for poor circulation, lessening blood clots, and edema, thus promoting the elimination of ama. Pungent is a taste not detectable according to Western concepts of digestive physiology. Pungent taste is prevalent in aromatic spices like ginger, cayenne, cardamom and mint. It is also in coffee and tea. Excessive use of these beverages may aggravate conditions described below.

Pungent taste taken too excessively causes burning sensation, dryness, weakness, fainting, tissue depletion, and can adversely affects the lungs and digestive tract. In moderation, pungent promotes proper weight, but excessive use will lead to congestion and constipation.

Astringent – This taste has a sedative and moderately cooling effect, moderately increases Vata, moderately decreases Pitta, and mildly decreases Kapha. It is anti-inflammatory and promotes vasoconstriction, stops diarrhea, reduces sweating, aids in healing, and promotes the clotting of blood. Astringent is another taste not recognized by Western concepts of physiology. It is experienced in tree bark and resin like myrrh and frankincense. It is also present in pomegranate, unripe banana and herbs such as turmeric, alum and goldenseal.

Astringent taste in excess causes contractions, muscle tension, constipation, obstructs speech by drying the mouth, and may increase Vata based nerve disorders such as numbness, spasms, and pain.

Tastes and the Doshas

Dosha	Mildly↓	Moderately↓	Strongly↓	Mildly↑	Moderately↑	Strongly↑
Vata	Sweet	Sour	Salty	Bitter	Astringent	Pungent
Pitta	Bitter	Astringent	Sweet	Sour	Pungent	Salty
Kapha	Pungent	Bitter	Astringent	Sweet	Salty	Sour

The best taste for Vata is sour.
The best tastes for Pitta are bitter and sweet.
The optimal tastes for Kapha are pungent and bitter.

Tastes and the Emotions

Yoga's purifying benefits increase when we begin to notice how our sensory organs influence our consciousness and moods. By paying attention to our multidimensional nature (described as the koshas), you can make yogic practice more profoundly effective. A major change occurs as we move from the first four stages of Ashtanga Yoga or the outer limbs to the fifth stage. The first four stages are concerned with physical activity; the fifth stage pratyahara has to do with the "appropriate use of senses and emotions." The Sanskrit word Rasa means both taste and emotion, implying an overlap of body and mind. Taste is to the body what emotion is to the mind.

In balance, tastes can produce harmonious emotions, but in excess, they can provoke negative tendencies. For example, in moderation sweet taste generates feelings of satisfaction and love. However, overly indulged in, sweetness can create feelings of greed and complacency. Salty taste shows a love of life and can be accompanied by an increase in all appetites. Yet salty taste in excess promotes hedonism and overindulgence. Sour generates desire for satisfaction and discernment but in extreme, it can lead to jealousy, envy and resentment. In balance, pungent taste results in stimulation, a craving for excitement, and extroversion; in excess it can promote irritability, criticism and hatred. Bitter taste can promote a positive desire to change for the best; overindulgence will increase feelings of frustration, grief and sorrow. Astringent taste promotes introversion, which can be helpful when life is too full. In excess, it can provoke insecurity and anxiety to a level that pushes the base emotion of fear into a state of panic.

Vata Pacifying Diet

As Vata tends to be the most readily imbalanced dosha, a Vata pacifying diet is needed more frequently than diets focused on other doshas. This is provided other influences such as seasonal weather patterns are minimally changed in your region. The following are some general recommendations by Dr. John Douillard for pacifying Vata. [43]

Favor foods that are warm, heavy, and oily. Focus on foods that are sweet (e.g., wheat, milk, rice), sour (e.g., yogurt, tomatoes, citrus fruit), and salty. Minimize foods that are cold, dry, and light. Avoid tastes of pungent (spicy), bitter (e.g., green leafy vegetables), and astringent (e.g., apples, beans).

I won't go into more specifics about diet or other dosha considerations as that has been covered more thoroughly in many Ayurvedic books.

VI. Yoga & Ayurvedic Purification Practices

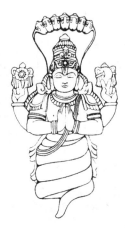

Ayurveda and Yoga view each individual as a unique whole, a solar system unto themselves. Like a solar system, people are influenced by changes in other parts of the universe, so that physical and spiritual health is constantly fluctuating. The goal of Ayurvedic Yoga Therapy is to be able to experience, perceive and understand not only how to adapt to change but also how to see through it to the spiritual constancy that lies behind it.

Yogic Purification Practices - Shatkarmas

The Six Purificatory Practices
"All the texts agree that pranayama is impossible
until the nerve channels (nadis) are thoroughly cleansed."[48]

The six purifications, Shatkarma Kriyas, are the methods of cleansing the gross channels (strotras) through which our physical and sensory nutrition pass. These gross channels interconnect with channels in the subtle body called nadis. The nadis are subtle tubes through which awareness flows. The Yoga texts describe ten major nadis. These channels end at the ten openings to the body – eyes, ears, nostrils, mouth, fontanel at the crown of the skull, urethra, and anus. The purification practices change internal pressures and heighten the capacity of the tubes to carry water, nutrients, waste products and sensory impressions. This will improve digestion and the functioning of all the senses. These Kriyas can also be used to re-direct attention inward away from the senses toward the threefold process of meditation called samyama in the Yoga Sutras, III, 4.

In the major classical Hatha Yoga texts, Hatha Yoga Pradipika II, 22-36 and the Gheranda Samhita I, 12-60, these cleansing practices are considered to be the "six purifiers of the bonds of karma." Before progressing to the more challenging practices of pranayama and prolonged meditation, it is important to increase one's vitality and solidify one's will, because without these, the deeper practices are unable to lead to transformative change. These practices can also help to create lifestyle changes leading to greater vitality and health. They are often therapeutic recommendations for those whose health needs to be restored.

The six practices consist of
1 - tratak, fixed gazing for purifying the eyes and lacteal glands;
2 - jala neti, water snuffing for cleansing the nostrils and sinuses;
3 - kapalabhati, "shining the skull," a breathing exercise for clearing the chest and upper lungs, thus reducing mucous and excess weight;
4 - dhouti, clearing of the upper intestinal tract;
5 - basti, enema for the health of the lower intestinal tract; and
6 - nauli for toning of the abdominal musculature and digestive organs, which can also increase sexual vitality.

Like many of the Classical Yoga techniques, they are best learned from an experienced teacher who knows how to practice them, and also how to adapt them to individual differences. Students are cautioned to seek a teacher trained in the methods to proceed beyond the basic instructions I have given here. Please follow the precautions noted as all practices challenge your ability to adapt your internal environment to a wide array of forces and manipulations. Each of these practices has a progression similar to that of pranayama, in that they move through the koshas from physical purification into the realm of heightening the body energy fields. At first pranayama is experienced as breathing exercises, exercises for the lungs and respiratory muscles; but with continued practice, students become adept at using pranayama to open the channels into the first layer of the energy body (Pranamaya kosha). This strengthens their emotional range and mental capacity. Initially, these practices purify the physical body of toxins and waste products; however, over time, they begin to work on a deeper level, and eventually pass through to the second layer of the subtle body (manomaya kosha), the source of thoughts. At this level they can help maintain a consistent, positive attitude. For example, fixed gazing (tratak) strengthens the ocular muscles and nerves then moves on to the process of withdrawal of the senses (pratyahara) and finally to an advanced technique called Shambhavi Mudra (see chapter on Pratyahara).

Precaution –

The Shatkriyas are strong purifiers of the internal systems, especially the nervous and digestive systems. You should increase your intake of fresh fruits and vegetables, ideally organic, being mindful to maintain a sense of balance, or irritability, moodiness, indigestion, constipation, or nausea may result. Ideally, if done correctly, you will notice an increasing sense of happiness, cheerfulness and positivity. If this is not the case, the purifications were not done properly – they may have been beyond your capacity, your preparations may have been inadequate, or you may have exceeded your body's rate of cleansing. If this is the case, seek experienced guidance before continuing further.

Fixed Gazing - Tratak

"Looking intently with an unwavering gaze at a small point until tears are shed, is known as tratak by the acharyas (master teachers). Tratak eradicates all eye diseases, fatigue and sloth and closes the doorway creating these problems." [49]

Of the numerous exercises used to prepare for deep meditation, fixed gazing (Tratak) produces the most profound benefit for the amount of time it takes to master this technique. Known in Yogic literature as a purifier (kriya) of the eyes and the lacteal glands, it also is a strengthening exercise for the eight eye muscles (located at the eye's four corners). With regular practice, Tratak also produces steadiness of the mind. Just as holding the body steady as a result of good asana practice enables one to more readily regulate the breath, so holding the gaze enables one to inwardly concentrate the mind.

Psychologists claim that 85% of our sensory input comes through visual awareness. Through this process, the practitioner becomes less distracted by the visual sense. In his book The Magical Child, Joseph Chilton Pearce cites that children will elicit this meditative state of expanded awareness naturally as they "sit motionless and gaze with a blank state", unless chastised by their parents for "spacing out." For the understanding parent, how wonderful it is for them to praise a child for possessing a natural introspection and taking a break from the sensory overload that characterizes our culture.

Precautions -

This practice is particularly beneficial for people who do not cry or who suffer from dry eyes. However, it would be best to blink frequently and moisten your eyes until your lacteal glands begin to produce more secretion. This technique trains you to be able to hold your eyes still, while relaxing your body, and is a great skill for developing openhearted communication in intimate relations, as eye movements reveal a tendency to hide feelings and thoughts. By being steady with your eyes, your mind will become steady and capable of "grasping onto the truth" (Gandhi's satyagraha). For no matter how intimate, fearful, or secretive the truth may be it always leads us to the highest course of activity (dharma). This is the powerful purification method that Gandhi used in securing India's independence.

Instructions -

To practice fixed gazing, begin by arranging your seat in a distraction free area that has a bare wall. Choose between sitting in a chair or on the floor. Of primary importance is to adjust your sitting posture to be comfortable and supportive of your back so you can remain stationary for 15 minutes. Then place a focalizing object in front of your seat at the level of your heart. The ideal object is one that you are readily attracted to. It could be a flower, a candle flame, a scene from nature, or the picture of a respected friend or teacher. Ideally it should be a minimum of elements so that your eyes will not be drawn to look at details. Once your focal area is arranged, close your eyes and take several deep breaths as you release any superficial tensions. Then gently open your eyes and gaze at the object, allowing your eyes to see it fully, but without attention to detail. Maintain an erect posture with natural breathing. Then just sit and watch.

Keep your eyes motionless as long as possible. If you need to blink, close your eyes for a moment then release the tension from your temples, jaws, and eyes with full audible exhales. Open your eyes and resume gazing. Start with five minutes without blinking, and gradually increase your gazing to 20-minutes without blinking. During this process there may be visual distractions – spots of colored light, haze over the object, streams of light, or hallucinations that produce distortions in the image. Just sit and allow these perceptions to arise. Allow your eyes and breath to remain soft, your lower jaw to remain relaxed. Tears may form, clouding your field of vision; just relax and briefly close your eyes. With persistence and a gentle sustained effort, it should take 3-4 weeks to master this level of practice.

With mastery of fixed gaze training, your eyes will deceive you less, and you will join Gandhi's peace troops as you learn to "hold onto the truth."

Variations

Another method is to gaze into a mirror placed at head level in a dark room so that only your face is visible. To achieve this, place a candle below your face so that only your face is lit. This practice is extremely powerful in overcoming fear, developing self-esteem, and courage. One is cautioned to not practice this until regular fixed gazing has been achieved for 20 minutes. The reason is that facial hallucinations can arise and frighten you. Sufficient courage and perseverance should be established before tackling this variation and looking to find the face of your true Self.

This process is particularly beneficial for those with substance addictions. Gaze at a picture of your addictive substance and train yourself to minimize your emotional and physical responses to it. Just see it as you would a candle flame or a flower. With time the charge of your addiction will be significantly reduced.

Benefits

This simple technique can have profound benefits including increased intuition and psychic sensitivity. It can also help to release suppressed emotions as it clears the channels for memory. Some students have reported insights into their early and past life relationships that brought about a greater ease in current life situations. It balances Alochaka Pitta.

Water Snuffing - Jala Neti

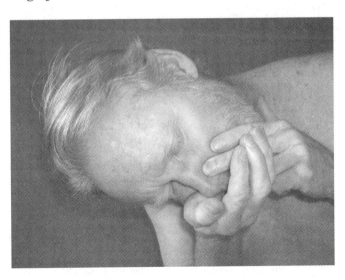

Neti cleanses the cranium and bestows clairvoyance. It also destroys all diseases that manifest above the throat." [50]

Nasal and sinus passages must be free of excess mucous in order to breathe freely. This practice is recommended for everyone contemplating pranayama, and it is mandatory for those engaged in a regular pranayama discipline. Mucous buildup restricts the passages making full respiration impossible. It also diminishes your sense of smell, which can interfere with memory. In yogic anatomy the senses each relate to an element. Earth element relates to smell. The easiest method for cleansing the nostrils is water snuffing (jala neti).

Precautions –
Water snuffing is exhilarating when performed properly. There are several guidelines that must be followed to prevent strains during your practice.It is important to carefully follow the instructions given as any variation can inflame your delicate mucosal respiratory lining. If the snuffing is done too strongly, or improperly, your eyes will water and your mucus membranes will feel strained.

Instructions -
Use the best water you can obtain. Some people find that using a half-teaspoon of sea salt per cup of water is more effective for removing excess mucous and allergens. As for myself I use only water. Fill the palm of your hand with lukewarm water, tilt your head to the right side, parallel to the floor, and remain in this position until you are done snuffing. Use your left hand to close off the upper nostril (left) and with a gentle snuff, draw the water into your lower right nostril and sinuses. Hold your head steady tilted to the side to allow the water to drain out of your nose and mouth. This should be practiced 3 times on each side, twice daily, either in your shower or following tooth brushing.

You can also use a clay neti pot to pour water directly into the upper nostril while leaning to one side. This effect is will be different, since the neti pot holds more water than the hand and you are relying on gravity to irrigate the upper nostrils and sinuses.

Benefits -
Water snuffing is an excellent process for deepening and stimulating Yoga pranayama. It helps to lessen pressure on the eyes, by keeping the sinus cavities open, free of congestion and airborne pollutants. It is particularly beneficial for people who are working in dusty or dirty areas, or who are sensitive to pollution. The more toxic your living or work environment, the more times you can do this per day.

Some of my students have claimed that they have seen major improvements in their chronic sinus conditions, postnasal drip, poor eyesight, and reduced headaches. It makes colds shorter and of a milder intensity. Instead of blowing your nose with tissue, practice water snuffing. More mucous is removed and the passages are left clearer for longer periods. By gradually training yourself to use cold water all year round it increases your immunity to seasonal colds and can lessen your reaction to allergens.

The range of benefits is large so I encourage you to give the practice a week of your time to discover what it has to offer you. This balances and purifies Tarpaka Kapha and lessens the tendency of Avalambaka Kapha to accumulate and form mucous in the head and chest.

Purifying the Breath - Kapalabhati

The term kapalabhati literally translates to the "head shining" practice. It is a breathing technique that, like water snuffing, clears your head and respiratory passages. Regular practice can create an aura of lightness, bring clarity to your mind, and relieve a number of conditions such as respiratory infections, eyestrain and allergies.

Precautions for this and the next two practices –

Kapalabhati, like all yogic abdominal cleansing practices, should not to be practiced by anyone with uncontrolled high blood pressure, pregnant or menstruating women, or people with heart conditions. It is best done one hour prior to a meal and at least two hours following a meal. It is imperative that the inward pull of the belly occurs only during exhalations; otherwise headaches and dizziness may result. Keep your upper body stationary without lifting your shoulders, tensing your neck, or dropping your chest. For the benefits to accrue the practice should be centered on the abdomen.

Instructions –

Water snuffing should precede kapalabhati, which should only be done in a stable, seated position. It consists of short, sharp abdominal contractions during each exhalation, at a stable rate of one per second, after which the air is inhaled without effort. Begin with a hand placed palm up upon your knee in Jnana Mudra (Wisdom Seal). Place your other palm on the middle of your abdomen. Begin with a natural breathing pace and make sure that your abdomen contracts away from your hand with each exhalation. After a minute begin to contract your navel more markedly on the exhalation while allowing your muscles to relax to normal position for the inhalation.

After the coordinated motion is maintained, you can begin to do the practice faster until the rate of 1 breath per second is established. Condition yourself to be able to reach the goal of 30 seconds of sustained practice. If the rhythm cannot be maintained then a shorter quantity can be done per round of practice.

Once the rhythm is sustained and motion is restricted to the abdomen, you can begin a formal round of practice, which consists of 30 breaths in thirty seconds. Breathe normally for 2-3 breaths, and then repeat the process for a second round. You can do up to three rounds of 30 breaths each provided your abdominal rhythm is steady. After completion, sit quietly and observe the effects of the practice. Allow your attention to be directed to what is a naturally arising point of concentration. Stay still for at least 3 minutes or go straight into your meditation practice from here.

Benefits

Regular practice reduces excess weight and balances Kledaka and Tarpaka Kapha. It also stimulates the digestive fire, Jatharagni, which may result in improved metabolism and improved elimination.

Cleansing the Digestive Fire - Agnisar Dhouti

The practitioners of Classical Yoga have raised cleansing the body to an art form. These methods are beneficial for all types of obstructions to or stagnation of the lubricating and digestive systems. The most familiar cleansing practices include showering, brushing the teeth, and removing wax accumulation from the ears. While these are common in most world cultures, this practice is unique to Classical Yoga.

Dhouti means, "to cleanse." The Gheranda Samhita I, 13 - 44 described four types of cleansing procedures – internal (antar-dhouti), teeth and face (danta-dhouti), esophagus (hrid-dhouti) and colon (sodhan-dhouti). There are four variations of internal cleansings for the digestive tract. They consist of cleansing with air, fire and two variations with water. Fire cleansing is the safest.

To a Yogini the abdominal region is the region of fire, and agnisar dhouti is the cleansing of the digestive fire. Health is the result of a healthy fire (Agni) which allows efficient digestion of food. This practice creates purification by increasing the movement of air in the fire region of the middle abdomen. This is the area that is responsible for maintaining a healthy core body temperature of 98.6° F. Imagine a fireplace with its firebox deep in your abdomen and its chimney rising up through your head. Let the pumping of your abdomen be like blowing into the firebox to intensify the combustion of the fire. Feel the heat in your deep abdomen increasing yet a mild portion of its warmth is spread upward to your heart and head.

Precautions –

The same considerations are here for this practice as the previous one – kapalabhati and the one to follow – nauli.

Instructions -

The best way to learn this practice is from a standing position. Prepare yourself by baring your abdomen so you can observe its movements throughout the practice. From this posture spread your feet slightly wider than hip distance and bend your knees. This will enable you to hold your torso still by placing your hands just above your knees with your arms straight. Tilt your head downward keeping your eyes open to watch your abdominal motions throughout the exercise. Inhale, relax your abdomen letting its contour fall forward with gravity, and then exhale pulling the central abdominal region backward. Repeat slow abdominal breathing three times, then inhale deeply and while exhaling lower your head until your chin is close to your chest in Jalandhara Bandha (neck lock). While restraining your breath, begin to pull back on your navel then relax it to normal position. Repeat the pull and relaxation of the central abdomen as many times as you can without breathing.

When you need to breathe take three full breaths allowing your abdomen to move in harmony with your breathing. This ends the first round. In between rounds do abdominal breathing until you feel rested. Then do two more rounds and count the number of pumps you can reach without getting out of breath. If you are exceeding your limit, you will gasp during the first breath following the pumping motions. The ideal is to have your breath come gently without any strain. A good goal to strive for is 30 pumps per round. Thus you will have a total of 90 pumps for the three rounds.

Benefits -
Regular practice increases the strength of your abdominals, and improves their stamina as it tones the diaphragm by increasing your breath holding time. This practice decreases Kledaka Kapha, increases Pachaka Pitta and Agni and therefore improves digestion. For students who are overweight, a consistent practice can help with weight loss.

Common Errors -
The pulling and releasing should be applied directly back and forth, unlike Udiyana Bandha, in which the pull is exerted back and upward, resulting in a hollow upper abdominal cavity. It is important to keep your head down both to maintain a neck lock, and to watch the motions to your central abdomen.

Variations -
Other variations of oral and facial dhouti include massaging the teeth and gums; cleansing the tongue and taste buds with a metal scraper or spoon; massaging and rinsing the outer ears to heighten hearing; and massaging the temples with the thumbs to improve eye sight, prevent cough, and soothe the nerves.

There are three variations for cleansing the esophagus - 1) with turmeric; 2) vomiting to remove bile; and 3) swallowing a ghee-lubricated cloth then slowly pulling it out to expel excess mucous. Therapeutic vomiting (Vamana dhouti), while sounding unpleasant, is highly beneficial in removing obstructive ama prevalent in chronic asthma and allergies. This practice is done first thing in the morning on an empty stomach. The previous night's dinner meal should be extra light. To do Vamana Dhouti make a solution of ½ teaspoon of sea salt per cup of water.

Then drink as much lukewarm saline water as you can tolerate or until there is a sensation of regurgitation. Bend forward from standing position over your toilet and allow the reflex to take over. If necessary, touch the uvula at the upper back of the throat to heighten the gag reflex.

Cleansing of the colon consists of both external and internal rectal massage with a lubricated finger to lessen tensions of the musculature of the pelvic floor and promote the flow of Apana Prana. This is also called Ganesh Kriya, named for the mythological elephant headed ruler of the third chakra. It is most beneficial in releasing deep-seated fear and/or to adjust a displaced coccyx (tailbone).

Tossing the Boat - Nauli

The word Nauli has its root in nau meaning boat and li meaning to toss, cling to, or lie on. One of my teachers referred to it as the "boat that you can cling to." In a sense life is a turbulent sea, and our body is a vessel; the purer the vessel, the more reliably it can weather the storms of life. This practice is unique in that no other form of exercise creates core tone by isolating the rectus abdominis muscles that lie in a central vertical line. The muscles attach just below the pectoral muscles of the chest and terminate in a narrow band at the upper section of the pubic bone. The rectus are paired muscles, one on either side of the navel, separated by a line of connective tissue or fascia called the linea alba, the "white line." The muscle is also divided into four vertical segments on either side. This muscle is responsible for the rippling effect (misnamed as "six packs" – actually there are eight segments) seen in highly toned slender athletes.   Once isolated, the rectus abdominis muscle appears like a thick rope or a vertical boat rising up from an abdominal sea.

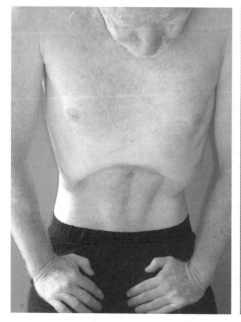 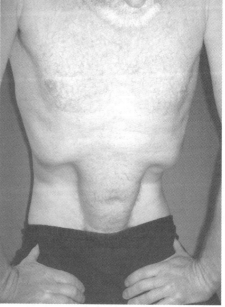

Precautions –

The same considerations are here for this practice as the previous two – kapal-abhati and agnisar dhouti.

Instructions -

In order to prepare for the practice, it is recommended that you be on a sat-tvic vegetarian diet for at least six months. This is a Kriya and it is important that you be committed to the process of cleansing your vessel. In addition, one needs to first master Agnisar Dhouti to a minimum of 100 pumps over four rounds and Stomach Lock (Uddiyana Bandha) held comfortably for a minimum of 20 seconds with three resting breaths in between four rounds. The Stomach Lock is an isola-tion of the diaphragm, which needs to be shown by a teacher who maintains a regular practice of these methods.

Begin by holding Uddiyana Bandha, then bring your hands to the tops of your thighs with your fingers turned inward so that your thumbs are hooked over the outer thighs. Strongly squeeze your upper thighs as you slowly release the stomach lock from the top to the bottom (see image on the left). By slowing the pace of the release your rectus abdominis muscle will naturally reveal itself isolated from the other abdominal muscles. The rectus will appear as two ropelike projections on either side of the hollow side muscles (see image on the right). Initially the formation of these hollow regions will create a vacuum that might cause you to loose your breath. Many students at this point will loose the grip of their Neck Lock. On future repetitions, concentrate on retaining your breath without force yet have a stronger Neck Lock that you can release slowly.

Once the middle (Madhya) Nauli is formed consistently, focus on developing the tone of the central muscles by narrowing their rope-like appearance. When you begin to feel the end of your breath retention capacity, release the pressure of your hands and the tension of your neck. Slowly inhale as you relax and gradu-ally fill your lungs from top to bottom creating the wave breath appearance on the surface of your abdomen. Take a minimum of three breaths to recover before repeating the procedure. Do no more than three repetitions. Once you have learned to isolate the central muscles focus upon developing their tone until they stand out more distinctly.

The second level of attainment is to move smoothly back and forth between Uddiyana Bandha and Nauli. Practice making the definitions of each muscle group, the diaphragm and the rectus abdominis, more distinct as you shift between the two techniques. Develop this tone until you can shift back and forth comfort-ably ten times on one breath.

To progress in your practice, develop your respiratory capacity by extending the breath pause time while maintaining a smooth release of Nauli. When you can complete three sets with three resting wave breaths then increase to four or five sets. Do not increase beyond nine sets interspersed with three wave breaths. If recovery takes more than three breaths you will be straining your internal organs, especially the heart muscle, from the profound vacuum created by this technique. Once you have gained sufficient stamina for nine rounds interspersed with three wave breaths, you can begin training for isolating each side of the rectus abdominis.

At this point, you are ready for the third level of practice. Shift the pressure of your hands off your left thigh while increasing the pressure on your right thigh. The increased pressure will tend to shift the rectus to the right. Avoid the tendency to shift your pelvis to the side. At the same time deepen the hollow on the left to help the muscle become more defined. Slowly release as before. Repeat on the opposite side. To develop your stamina use the same training sequence as for the middle Nauli. With regular practice you can begin to roll the muscles from side to side. This rolling will appear like the rope rolling across the front surface of your abdomen.

The most advanced level of practice will come by shifting the rolling into a circular clockwise then counterclockwise motion. This will give the appearance of a rope fixed at the ceiling being moved in a circle from someone manipulating the lower attachment. In this method, the rectus is moved from forward left to right then to the back right then back left, then forward left again. Take several resting breaths then reverse the flow to make the circle move counterclockwise. Once these motions are complete without strain, Nauli has been mastered.

Common Errors include –
- Not fully extending your spine and retaining the lift of your rib cage.
- Looking elsewhere, lifting your head and loosing Jalandhara Bandha
- Loosing the breath, either due to inadequate relaxation in the intervals between exertions or the capacity to maintain natural breath suspension is not developed.
- Nausea - doing the practice without an empty stomach
- Coming erect as a result of Uddiyana Bandha and attempting Nauli with straight legs.
- Pushing the pelvis to one side in an attempt to develop the weaker side or to isolate one half of the rectus abdominis muscle.

Benefits –
This practice helps to increase Agni and balance Pitta. It provides similar benefits to Uddiyana Bandha as it also increases abdominal tone, reduces fat and increases respiratory capacity. It is the most advanced practice for toning the digestive and respiratory muscles. Many students who have strong lungs from running or swimming are surprised at how difficult it is to master this exercise. It is often added as part of a therapeutic program for asthma. The practice squeezes the blood and nutrients into each tissue and organ while aiding in the expulsion of waste matter. For this reason, it is beneficial in situations where the liver and/or pancreas have been threatened from a high sugar diet or from abuse of alcohol.

After 3-6 months of consistent practice, students have reported a decrease of symptoms of constipation, prolapse of the uterus, irritable bowel syndrome, colitis, menstrual irregularities, incontinence, impotence and premature ejaculation.

Cleansing the Colon - Basti

Basti has two forms dry (sthala) and wet (jala). Both practices require the mastery of asanas, the ability to remain motionless in the required asanas for a minimum of three minutes while holding a firm Mula Bandha. In addition, the student needs to be in a steady pose prior to applying abdominal muscle isolations (Agnisar Dhouti, Uddiyana Bandha, and Nauli). Until sufficient practice is achieved for isolation with each technique, the integration of all the asanas, bandhas, and dhouti necessary for this practice will not grant full benefits.

Precautions -
Begin slowly, starting with the dry technique and then proceeding to the water enema. Be gentle not to strain your breath during retentions.

Instructions -
For the dry version of the practice, Sthala Basti, choose between two postures Westside Back Stretch (Paschimottanasana) or Inverted Action (Viparita Karani Mudra). I recommend starting with the inverted posture as it is somewhat easier to retain the water in this pose. The practice involves the use of churning the abdomen (as in Agnisar Dhouti) and repetitive anal contractions and relaxations (Aswini Mudra). When practiced properly this method will bring air in and out of the rectum and help promote peristalsis for free motion of the contents of the colon.

Variation - Water Enema -
Jala Basti (Yogic water enema) is a more advanced practice, as it requires the mastery of Uddiyana Bandha and Nauli. It is traditionally practiced while squatting in a stream or ocean so that the water level is above the waist. However, it is more suitable to practice in the privacy of your bathroom. Begin by standing in a half squatting posture with your knees bent and hands around lower thighs. In this position practice Stomach Lock, and as you release it let go of all the air inside the abdominal and pelvic cavities. Do several repetitions to insure your abdomen is relaxed and receptive to changes in circulation.

Then take a pint or up to a quart of water into the rectum through a warm water douche while lying on your left side. Return to a standing half squat position and hold the water inside through a strong steady Mula Bandha. Then do Nauli to pull the water more interiorly. Through this method a vacuum is created inside the colon that allows the water to be drawn upwards. The next level of mastery involves moving the water higher into the transverse colon, by the side-to-side motions of Nauli.

Then sit on the toilet and release the water, discharging it from your colon. A more ideal posture is to go into a full squatting position with feet only a few inches below the pelvis. In India toilets are on the floor, which enables a full evacuation of the colon, from being in a full squat. Then expel all the contents of the colon by rapidly contracting and releasing the anal sphincter, this will expel the water in spurts. This technique is called Horse Seal (Aswini Mudra). Repeat until all the water is expelled. Follow the procedure by taking a rest with a long Corpse Pose (Savasana) of at least 20 minutes.

Ayurvedic Purification Practices – Panchakarmas

Ayurveda has similar practices to the Yogic Kriyas done in five parts. Panchakarma can accomplish many things for the body: langhana (reducing), brhana (nourishing), shodhana (purifying it of ama or residues), and shamana (pacifying doshas).

The goal of Ayurvedic treatment is to restore balance between the individual's current status, Vikruti, and their primary constitution, Prakruti. According to this perspective, illness results from the aggravation of doshas, which leads to chronic imbalances. Ayurveda's goal is to create, and as far as possible, sustain serenity in the agitated dosha. For instance, if Vata is aggravated, it may produce symptoms in different sites such as constipation, dull pain, dry cough, headache, and restlessness. While each dosha has a main region and home organ, they are pervasive throughout the body; so that each dosha can produce symptoms in any organ or tissue. Regardless of the imbalance, balancing Vata and returning the pranas to their home region and function can rectify most symptoms even when diffuse. Thus while different procedures may be warranted for different individuals, all students need to have a sadhana that begins and concludes with Vata balancing.

Both Yoga and Ayurveda see the need for purification techniques that improve our ability to sustain health and increase the efficacy of our eliminative organs. These procedures are used in Ayurvedic clinics with special diets, Yoga practices, and massage. In an ideal clinical environment, they would be administered daily for a 1-6 week period and personally adapted for each client. They are helpful both as a preventive procedure as well as treatment for acute and chronic symptoms of dosha imbalances. Normally two procedures are given in the days preceding the Panchakarma procedure; they are massage with medicated oils (Snehana) and sweating (Swedana) to increase the elimination of wastes through the skin. As the skin is the largest organ of elimination, increasing the health of their pores is a natural way to bring toxins out from deeper tissues into the skin and hollow organs for elimination. These two procedures make one feel wonderful and many day spas and clinics offer only the preliminary methods, as they are not equipped with residential facilities necessary for the complete process.

This preliminary procedure helps the digestive, eliminative and sensory organs to function at peak efficiency. Once this has been successfully accomplished, then the rest of the purification procedures can be utilized effectively. The five Ayurvedic procedures are upper digestive tract cleansing (Vamana), medicated purgation (Virechana), therapeutic blood letting (Rakta Mokshana), enema (Basti), and nasal medications (Nasya). Purgation is especially for treating imbalances in Pitta and Kapha, blood letting for Pitta, upper digestive tract cleansing for Pitta and Kapha, enema for Vata, and nasal medication for Vata. The last three methods are similar to three of the six methods of Yoga's cleansing repertoire.

Ayurveda's purification practices are concerned with the removal of obstructed doshas as a preventative treatment as well as therapeutic application for treatment of specific diseases. It is felt that when preventative treatment is given, the tendency for the imbalances to form ama can be eliminated. These practices are different for various seasons. Fall and spring are the seasons best suited for treating Vata. Medicated enemas and nasal medications are best utilized during this season. Fall and spring are also the periods for reducing excess and imbalanced Kapha, more deeply cleansing the upper gastrointestinal tract, through purgation. Summer is the season for treating imbalances in Pitta. Practices of therapeutic cleansing of the upper digestive tract, bloodletting, and purgation are used then. Since these procedures are to be administered to your clients rather than a practice for yourself, my descriptions of them will be brief. Once they have been experienced the student can progress to learning how to personally adapt the methods for personal application.

Emotional Release

The cleansing practices of Ayurveda and Yoga often bring out a discharge of suppressed emotions held in the physical tissues or subtler koshas. The chest and mucous linings of the upper digestive tract and the respiratory tract are often filled with incomplete emotional experiences. This is one of the major reasons why these procedures are not recommended to be given to yourself. This is especially true in the cases where one is clearing out long standing suppressed emotions, physical congestion, or diseases of the upper body.

The Ayurvedic practitioner can guide the client in expressing their emotions and remaining as physically relaxed as possible so the feelings do not find other tissues to suppress them. Ayurvedic and Yoga Therapists need to be clear of the emotional areas that may arise or there will be transference or projection of stress from client to therapist. They need to develop a solid referral network with holistic therapists grounded in meditation and spiritual practices who can assist in the deep purifications.

Kapha discharges will often be strong, vocal and may involve the use of shoulder and arm motions. Clients need to be given a free space perhaps even on the floor to discharge these most deeply seated emotions of attachment. Often insights will arise about situations that could have eliminated the suffering of themselves or others. With this insight may also come self criticism.

Pitta predominant people most commonly experience their emotional discharge as criticism; in extreme cases, anger and violent images in dreams may seek expression before they are eliminated. Clients with a history of difficult emotions may find that they become serene, detached from their emotional disturbances.

Vata predominant clients will discharge feelings of fear and confusion. Once the suppressed emotions are expressed, the client can then experience profound relaxation, release of deep-seated primal fears, and an increased ability to enjoy sensory pleasures.

Medicated Nasal Cleansing - Nasya

This procedure is used for cleaning accumulated doshas in the throat, nasal and sinus passages. It is also used for treating overly stimulated senses, calming the mind and for neurological conditions affecting the sensory and motor functions. It is also used for problems related to the perception of sight, sound, and smell; and in some cases, even epilepsy, migraines, and respiratory difficulties. As Adya Prana predominates in this region, this Prana will be most affected by this procedure.

The procedure often begins with nasal massage using ghee and specialized herbs inserted by the little finger. A gradual deepening of the massage is done to assist in freeing tissue obstructions that may be present due to a deviated septum or incorrect alignment of the facial and cranial bones. The client is encouraged to breathe normally allowing the mixture to circulate through the nasal passages. Follow-up treatments will utilize various aromatic or detoxifying herbs. One mixture using calamus and ghee is called the Yogi's snuff as it assists in opening the third eye to develop spiritual visions and intuition.

Therapeutic Vomiting - Vamana

The preliminary methods will have brought obstructions and ama to the upper channels of elimination where Vamana can be used to remove them from the upper body.

Unlike the Yogic procedure that uses only water, in this method typically a mixture of calamus, licorice and honey is used to cleanse the chest, stomach, and nasal passages.

Medicated Purgation - Virechana

This procedure is for cleaning accumulations of toxic Pitta and Kapha through the lower body. Different preliminary procedures are given to move the obstructions into the lower digestive tract. The main action of the purgatives or laxatives chosen is to be upon the small intestine. One common formula is a mixture of triphala, powder from senna leaves, rhubarb, and castor oil.

Medicated Enema - Basti

There are many different procedures for cleansing the lower digestive tract, one of which is enemas. In a basic enema warm soapy water is used to cleanse the descending colon, the upper reaches of the next segment, the transverse colon, and even the last section, the ascending colon. Variations include decoction enema which is given in a dose of one-quart mixture of honey, rock salt and water; and oil enema which uses ghee or other oils with a mixture of medicinal herbs. The client lays on a slant board to allow the solution to be introduced into the anal canal and abdominal massage is sometime used to assist the mixture in moving upward.

Blood Letting - Rakta Mokshana

Waste products of digestion circulate through the blood stream and may become caught in capillaries in discolored veins of the hands and feet or around larger joints. In some cases of Pitta derangement of the spleen, skin, and liver, this procedure is beneficial. Though it is not beneficial where there is chronic weakness or anemia. This procedure is especially purifying for Pachaka Pitta. This technique is rarely done in America, as the practitioner in most states must be a licensed physician or acupuncturist to perforate the skin.

An easy way to practice this technique is to donate blood. It is beneficial to menopausal women, as it may aid in the adjustment to loosing their monthly cycle. The passing of the pint of blood required for donation acts much like menstruation and may sustain balance in Ranjaka and Pachaka Pitta. It also elevates the ojas quality of Kapha dosha as by selflessly giving to another we don't even know, it opens our hearts.

Eye Exercises

These supplemental Yoga exercises are for strengthening the eye muscles and purifying the optic nerves. The effects are more profound than Fixed Gazing, which should be mastered first. This series should be sequenced after the Joint Freeing poses or Pavanmuktasana, described in <u>Structural Yoga Therapy</u>. Begin sitting in Easy pose (Sukhasana) with your eyes closed. Steady your breathing until your inhale and exhale are of even duration. Concentrate on holding your body motionless, particularly your head. When stillness and comfort have been attained, open your eyes and gaze softly straight ahead in the following ways –

1. DISTANT TO CLOSE: Sit in front of a window that affords the greatest distant view possible. Slowly move your focus to closer and progressively closer objects until your attention is three feet ahead. Then place your forefinger at eye level and gaze at the tip of that finger. Slowly move your hand inward until your fingertip is resting on the tip of your nose. Reverse your visual focus until you are looking at the distant horizon. Repeat three times.

2. SIDE TO SIDE: Move your eyes in a straight line to the far right without moving your body. Keep your eyes focused, noting the farthest point that you

can see without distortion. Then move your eyes in a smooth steady line to the left, again finding the most distant focal point without turning your head. Repeat 3x each direction, then close and relax your eyes.

3.   TOP TO BOTTOM: Move your eyes up to the highest focal point then down to the lowest focal point, without moving your head.   Repeat 3x, then close your eyes and rest them.

4.   DIAGONAL: Look up and to the right, at a 45-degree angle. Move your eyes in a diagonal line opposite lower corner. Repeat 3x, and then rest your eyes. Then do the same exercise beginning at upper left moving to lower right. Repeat 3x.

5.   CIRCLES: Open your eyes, focusing at top center and slowly moving in a smooth clockwise manner to the extreme of each focal point. Repeat 3x. Close your eyes for one complete breath then repeat 3x counterclockwise.

6.   PALMING: Close your eyes and rub your palms briskly together until they become warm. Place your palms directly over the eyes with your fingers in you hair. Do not touch your eyelids but cup your hands close enough to feel the warmth of your palms. Your hands should be placed in such a manner as to shut out all light. Then open your eyes and focus on the blackness so your muscles and optic nerves obtain a deep rest.   Direct the Adya prana into its subtler form as vyana prana. This change will permit you to shift from being receptive to sensory input to perceptive to intuition.

This exercise is one of the best methods for relieving eyestrain and securing relaxation to improve eyesight. If it is difficult to "see" blackness with your eyes closed then lay a piece of black felt, velvet, or black "sleep mask" over your eyes after palming. An ideal tool for this purpose is an eye bag made of silk with rice or flax seed inside, scented or not, available in most health food stores. This is done while lying supine in the yoga relaxation exercise called Savasana.

1.   "When palming is perfect, the color of any object remembered is remembered perfectly and one feels perfectly relaxed and sees a perfect black field before the eyes when they are closed and covered.

2.   When the eyes are opened, perfect sight comes instantaneously and the letters on the eye chart seem perfectly black and are easily recognized.

3.   The white centers of the letters called halos seem to be whiter than the margin of the chart." [51]

VII. Ayurvedic Perspective on Yoga Poses

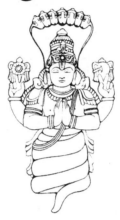

The Varieties of Yoga

To a beginner seeking to learn Yoga, confusion arises in searching for a class, as there are several forms of Yoga promoted in America. Rarely do we see physical Yoga referred to in its generic traditional name, Hatha Yoga. Instead, we are faced with a multitude of other brand names that are used to distinguish one methodology from the others. Some are based on a creative teacher's names like Iyengar Yoga, Kripalu Yoga, Bikram Yoga, and Sivananda Yoga. Others are based on the unique methods emphasized like Power Yoga, Ashtanga Yoga, Jivamukti Yoga, Viniyoga, or Tri Yoga.

In truth, all these are varieties of the generic term Hatha Yoga in that they focus the students practice primarily on limb three (asana) of Patanjali's Classical Yoga eight limb method. A few of them incorporate some aspects of the fourth limb (pranayama) and beyond into meditation. When they are approached with discrimination and guided by committed teachers, these styles all have wonderful health benefits to offer students.

Let us consider the major types of Yoga from an Ayurvedic perspective. Three popular teaching styles promoted as Kripalu Yoga, Integral Yoga and Sivananda Yoga are fairly similar in that they emphasize the use of rhythmic breathing, varieties of pranayama and mindfulness meditation practices while performing the yoga poses. The asanas are presented in a manner that is a preparation for the deeper practices of meditation. These wonderful practices make the body supple and the mind alert. It appeals to students who want to relax, change the pace of their lifestyle, and receive intuitive guidance in the direction their life needs to move. It is especially beneficial for those under going stress, mid life crisis, or seeking transition to a different vocation. This style is most ideal for those with a Vata predominant constitution. Making a commitment to any of these styles will assist the student in consistently balancing their Vata dosha.

A second category of Yoga presentations is Bikram Yoga, Power Yoga and Ashtanga Yoga that emphasize fast paced practices that are vigorous, aerobic in nature, and promote sweating as a form of purification. The practices develop lustrous skin tone, tremendous vitality, and a passion for life awakens. It is quite popular among American city-dwelling young professionals. These students find it suitable for their face-paced high demand lifestyle. This style is ideal for students with a Pitta predominant constitution, provided that they use their discernment and not get too heated up. These styles would not be recommended for a Pitta predominant student lacking discrimination in following their own guidance. However, for a balanced Pitta, this style will promote insight by keeping them engaged in the art of balancing and directing their fiery nature. They develop the most athletic bodies of all the types of Yoga.

The third style, Iyengar Yoga, is focused on physical alignment and the development of mental and physical strength and stamina. Once the basics have been learned, the teachers encourage holding the postures for long periods of time.

However, sometimes a beginning student will complete only four or five poses in a 90-minute class, and loose the benefit of a challenge to their physique. In this method, stamina and strength are emphasized. The practitioners become strong with moderately developed physiques. The emphasis is upon being firm and steadfast in the practice of asana. Faith and perseverance are developed by this beautiful method. This style is beneficial for those with a predominantly Kapha constitution. Viniyoga and the teachings of Prof. Krishnamacharya and his son Desikachar emphasize adapting the programs to individual needs and are more aligned with Classical Yoga and Ayurvedic guidelines. This method is primarily taught individually, rather than in group classes. While this method is primarily for Vata balancing, it can be suitable for any of the doshas, provided the instructor has been trained in Ayurvedic principles.

In this book we will draw from the foundational guidelines of Ayurveda encouraging the principles that will balance each dosha rather than focus on any one particular school of Yoga.

Ayurvedic Guidelines for Exercise

The Ayurvedic text, <u>Caraka Samhita</u> does not comment on Yoga asanas but it does offer advice about exercise in general. The aphorisms given are in Chapter VII: "31 - Such a physical action, which is desirable and is capable of bringing about bodily stability and strength is known as physical exercise. This has to be practiced in moderation. 32 - Physical exercise brings about lightness, ability to work, stability, resistance to discomfort and alleviation of doshas (especially Kapha). It stimulates the power of digestion. . . . Perspiration, enhanced respiration, lightness of the body, inhibition of the heart and such other organs of the body are indicative of the exercise being performed correctly. . . 36 - Exercise is contra-indicated for persons who are emaciated due to excessive sexual activity, weight lifting, and by traveling on foot and for those who are in the grip of anger, grief, fear, exhaustion, and for children, for old persons and for persons having Vata constitution and profession of speaking too much. One should not do exercise while he is hungry and thirsty also." [52]

Vata predominant people tend to be in constant motion, fidgeting, adjusting their spine, and rarely still. For them, exercise needs to be deliberate and conscious; done in coordination with breathing to hold their wandering mind. Rhythmic exercise, done regularly will be most helpful. They do not need a long program only one that is captivating, with plenty of attention to detail yet progressively taking them into themselves. They need to avoid being adjusted too much in classes by their teachers as this will promote instability. They will benefit greatly by taking the time at the end of class to thoroughly relax and meditate, even after others are packing up their mats.

Pitta predominant students do well with vigorous exercise that challenges their love of competition and assertiveness. Best are team activities that allow them cooperation and sharing of their skills. They will also do well in competitions against themselves. Yoga can be done in a fiery manner yet they need to learn to hold themselves back and develop discernment about how much to push themselves. If they find that they are developing Pitta conditions of increased heat then they will benefit greatly by taking some time off and swimming to reduce their propensity to increased fire. They can easily be aggravated into progressive degenerative conditions like arthritis.

Kapha predominant students need to exert themselves more than the other doshas. They need to develop a regular routine of exercise yet it should not become too habitual. Activities that are done in the same manner like bicycling, rowing, and running are not as beneficial for them. They do best with complicated routines that challenge their ability to stay present and physically challenging programs that build their cardiovascular health. Instead, they can do cross-country running where the courses and pace are varied. They need to watch themselves for the tendency to accumulate excess mucous or tissue. These are signs that a cleansing diet or more mentally and physically challenging exercise program is warranted.

For all forms of exercise according to a leading exponent, Dr. Svoboda "Ayurveda's rule is that you should never exert more than half your capacity." [53] Dr. Svoboda seems to have adapted this guideline from Caraka Samhita VI, 31 quoted previously. This moderation in exercise is aligned with Patanjali's axiom in Yoga Sutras II, 47 to "relax your effort" during asana practices in order to perfect your practices so that your experience moves in alignment with the progression delineated in Patanjali's text.

Dr. Svoboda is the first Westerner to complete Ayurvedic medical training in India. I have found that his perspective to be the most helpful in interpreting Ayurveda to our western mentality and lifestyle. I highly recommend his writings. Another helpful interpretation he has given comes from his Tantrik spiritual teacher, Vimalananda who "used to say that even if you ignore all other rules of routine, you can still maintain good health as long as you:
Keep your bowels moving (keep your colon clean)
Keep your body moving (exercise regularly)
Keep your breath moving (always breathe slowly and deeply)." [54]

Yoga asanas are a sub-category of the general physical actions cited by Caraka. His guidelines are relevant to all forms of movement – dance, competitive sports, weekend athletics, aerobics, or more passive exercises suchas computer games. When these guidelines are followed, exercise promotes health and a clear mind. In addition to the benefits cited, Yoga exercises when practiced according to the guidelines of Patanjali's Classical Yoga, creates a transformation of the mind. Classical Yogasana practice following Patanjali's Yoga Sutra guidelines, progressively leads the Yogini through a series of steps culminating in being free from the dualistic nature of mind/body that is the gross root of all conflicts.

Integrating Yogasana and Ayurveda

The Ayurvedic and Yogic traditions hold different but mutually supporting roles for each other. Ayurvedic guidelines help to create the lifestyle and understanding of the external world necessary to support and preserve health. Yogic guidelines support the spiritual perspective revealing that there is more to life than health, financial success, and family life. They constantly remind the student of the importance of meditation and prayer as the primary means of developing contact with Spirit as the means to contentment. In the development of Yogasana, Patanjali presents the importance of the spiritual perspective.

II, 46
Yoga pose (asana)
is a steady
and comfortable position.

II, 47
Yoga pose is mastered
by relaxation of effort,
lessening the natural tendency
for restlessness,
and identification
of oneself as living
within
the infinite stream of life.

II, 48
From that
perfection of yoga posture,
duality,
such as praise and criticism,
ceases
to be a disturbance. [55]

The classical definition of Yogasana, sukham sthiram asanam, as translated above II, 46 is known by all serious students of Yoga. The importance of preserving comfort and stability for the body in any position, regardless of the phase of life we live in, is assumed. I often like to twist this sutra by reflecting that Yoga Therapy is the removal of the causes of discomfort and instability. When approached in this manner, asana can be a great boon in applying its principles to achieve harmony in daily activities.

Selective Relaxation

The next sutra (II, 47) revels how to move toward mastering of asana. This sutra provides profound insight in how to practice Yogasana for optimal benefits. The first phrase of the sutra "relaxation of effort" can be seen as a parallel to the process Herbert Benson, MD describes as the <u>Relaxation Response</u>.[56] This Relaxation Response is a natural physiological phenomenon, Dr. Benson described as a parasympathetic reflex that he used in developing therapies for many stress-induced illnesses. I worked at the Mind Body Medical Institute in Boston, founded by Herbert Benson, MD and Dr. Joan Borysenko, for five years. Their strategy is highly parallel to that described by Patanjali two millennia ago. The process he described in his book consists of four steps:

1 - A quiet environment free of internal and external distractions
2 - A comfortable position, consciously relaxing the body's muscles
3 - A mental device that reflects your deepest personal beliefs
4 - A passive attitude toward intrusive thoughts

From the yogic point of view, the fourth step in this process is applied as a technique called Selective Relaxation. While doing a Yogasana, it is integral to Patanjali's guidelines to consciously lessen the effort involved in all activities. Physiological studies have confirmed what intuition tells us to be true – adept athletes are more efficient at using their bodies than novices. Adepts use less muscular tension and are more effective in their activity. Novices are more prone to getting injured, stressed, tense and fatigue easier than adepts do. This is true for all activities. Learning how to practice with less muscular effort can allow a typist to perform better, longer. In the same manner, the yogi can do more complex positions and actually become refreshed rather than tired by the activity.

On a practical note, Selective Relaxation consists of several phases of development. The first level of training is to learn to perform the positions without pain. At this level, the student gains discrimination between the spectrum of effort that goes from feeling the effort to strain and pain. There is clearly to be effort during Yogasana. Otherwise, Patanjali would not have used the phrase "relaxation of effort." His choice of words is always precise. This first level of introspection makes possible a perspective of asana as an inner task, rather than an external form to be achieved. For many students, this is a battle to constantly engage in as the mind struggles for self centered, ego validation. To shift gears from the apparent cultural values of "more is better" may not set well with some students. They will continue to push themselves hard, to apply competitive goal toward more flexibility, strength or "picture perfect" Yogasana practice.

The mental shift Yogasana is encouraging is subtle, yet producing major impact upon the attitude that drives all your life activities. It is among the crucial pivotal points in distinguishing Yoga from competitive sports like gymnastics. Some contemporary Yoga schools have gone so far from the classical teachings as to promote Yoga competitions with scoring for "perfect asanas" based on Olympic competition guidelines for gymnastic floor exercises. As Nischala Devi, author of The Healing Path of Yoga, put it, "Yoga is popular but what is popular is not Yoga." To stay on track so that you achieve the serenity and health goals defined by Patanjali, it is crucial that you do the practices following the Yoga Sutra guide-lines. Find a teacher trained in this method if you wish to go deep.

This first level of Selective Relaxation is the place where we can apply Yoga principles to daily tensions from situations where we are working too hard, strug-gling to have things go our way. This gross level of stress responds well to the application of sutra II, 47. It is not for those who are stress free beings but for the majority of the world. It is both preventative maintenance revealing our tendencies towards agitation and for those other times when we are markedly agitated.

Secondly, students are asked to feel within themselves how much they are ef-forting. This often produces the question in some students of where should I feel it? Am I doing it correctly if I feel it where I do? There is an answer to these questions, as an aligned adept will feel the sensations of specific muscles stretching or toning during each Yogasana. This is defined in the Asana Kinesiology chart in my book, Structural Yoga Therapy.[57] The line of inquiry into where you experi-ence the effort is highly relevant for those students in pain. They need to learn what sensations to encourage and what to discourage so that their bodies do not create more pain, but comfort. For the healthy student, this line of inquiry is only beneficial in learning physical anatomy. While this is a wonderful endeavor to pursue, learning anatomy and its application to motion, kinesiology, is not needed for the experiences defined in these sutras of Classical Yoga. Here, we are going beyond the scope of this more foundational level of training, so these questions are irrelevant to the student's progression.

This is a sidestep from Patanjali's more direct line of inquiry into simply feeling your effort in the asana and relax it to the point that you can remain comfortable and steadfast. For me, the subjective level Patanjali is seeking is to use 70% of your effort's capacity. At full effort, there is excess physical energy being misdirected. At this level, muscles are at odds with each other. While learning anatomy can facilitate clarity of understanding the function, it is intention that actually directs our movements. Through an intention to relax and steady our effort, the mind is freed to create detachment from the body's activities. Only a subtle detachment is required to feel beneath the waves of the multitude of bodily sensations. This moves the Yogi's attention to the subtler dimensions of being. Our musculo-skel-etal system comprises about 60% of our body's mass, so learning from their mes-sages is a crucial step of self-observation along the path to self-knowledge. Their messages consist of "currents of sensation" that are potential intuitive teachings that discernment training can translate into words. With sensitivity to repeated patterns of personal tension, the intention to relax and become comfortable with this subtle body language will manifest.

In this progressive manner, objective experience of steadiness is coupled with subjective training; forever deepening relaxation and comfort. The Yogasana is a vehicle for learning Selective Relaxation to "create a lessening of the natural tendency for restlessness." This training is central to the establishment of freedom from stress. Selective Relaxation is the process of learning to utilize your body's energies in a personal sense of ecology. Tension and effort is applied only to those areas necessary to create and sustain a position. All other muscles are consciously relaxed. This relaxation especially applies to the neck, face and respiratory muscles. The tension is not intended to be complete but rather partial and selective. When learned, the internal organs, nerves and cardiovascular system benefit tremendously. The training is heightened during the process of Progressive Relaxation (usually given at the final fifteen minutes of a Yoga class). Through this method, the layers of chronic tension are released, freeing up the creative mind.

The third step in the process of Selective Relaxation is "to lessen the natural tendency for restlessness." By becoming aware of the body, there may arise the perception that some sort of adjustment is necessary (especially for students with excessive and/or imbalanced Vata). As students feel their body's messages, they are often flooded with a stream of communication that has been backed up by being on vacation from attending to their body's messages. Not unlike our experience of taking a vacation to a tropical site and returning to an enormous pile of snail mail and email correspondence. Priority must be established in order to re-enter the former life in a gentle way. In the same manner, some body messages do not need attention at all and we can deal with them like we would junk mail and disregard from them. Other sensations need immediate attention or dis-ease will ensue. This step of Selective Relaxation is about choice and discernment. Choosing to keep a certain level of effort, a familiar wave of breath motion and e-motion (energetic or emotional motion) in the body/mind that allows the student to feel they are on familiar ground though not necessarily at peace with themselves.

The final phase of Patanjali's sutra on mastery of body pose talks of "identification of oneself as living within the infinite stream of life." This is a shift to the underlying awareness that is constantly within us. The image spoken of by Patanjali is that of the Lord of the Self, is reclining on the back of a snake (ananta), which in turn is floating on the sea of Life. This image is one of being at ease in spite of the constancy of life's changes. The Life Force is constantly moving requiring us to perpetually adapt to change. We do it all the time, sometimes without complaining and sometimes with resentment. These are the surface waves that Yoga can help us to be in right relationship with. To learn to respond where appropriate and to learn detachment in situations that are best left in others or God's hands. This of course takes practice and develops with the maturity of our spiritual evolution as well as our chronological evolution. Perhaps when we finally grow up, we will ride the waves of our Life with more grace.

As in all other aspects of the eight limbs of Classical Yoga, Patanjali gives us a clue to know if our training is complete in this step. His final sutra on asana II, 48 states "from that perfection of yoga posture, duality ceases to be a disturbance."

This is a tremendous statement. This is one of the hallmarks of a Yoga master. If you want to know if your teacher has achieved mastery, just watch and see how free from disturbance they are.

In Classical Yoga, the malleability of your physical body has little or nothing to do with mastery. Yoga adepts are those whose bodies and minds are free from the influences of the currents of sensation. In others, these sensations create responses of fear, anxiety, lethargy, and are in some fashion translated as stress and suffering. In contrast, a master chooses what to respond to; they are not victims of external or internal stimuli.

Yoga masters know a happiness
that is independent of circumstances.

Classifications of Yoga Poses

Yoga postures can be classified according to the features that they resemble or seek to evoke. When Yoga practice is done in a Tantrik perspective, they can produce a shamanic doorway to experiencing the individual components of the external world within yourself. The Tantrik perspective was born in the middle ages. Among its prime directives is that "Whatever is outside is inside. Whatever is not outside is not inside." Here are some of the qualities and attainments that Tantrik Yogis have gained.

Names of animals (Cobra - Bhujangasana, Crocodile - Makarasana, Fish - Matsyasana)

Names of sages (Siddhasana, Vasisthasana, Bharadvajasana)

Names of qualities (Warrior – Virabhadrasana, Hero – Virasana)

States of life (Fetal - Garbhasana, Corpse - Savasana)

According to body parts (Shoulder pose – Kandarasana; Shoulderstand – Sarvangasana; Headstand – Sirsasana)

Names of nature (Tree – Vrksasana; Lotus – Padmasana)

Geometrical figures (Triangle – Trikonasana; Circle/Wheel – Chakrasana)

Asanas can be classified in six different ways depending upon the effects that they produce.

1. Those that work on the spinal column:
   (Cobra - Bhujangasana, Bow - Dhanurasana, Locust - Salabhasana, and Fish - Matsyasana).

2. Those that work on the muscles of the extremities:
   (Face of Light - Gomukhasana, Eagle -Garudasana, and Warrior - Virabhadrasana).

3. Those that work on the hollow organs in the chest and abdomen:
   (Wind Freeing Pose - Apanasana, Fetal - Garbhasana, and spinal twists such as Marichyasana and Matsyendrasana).

4. Those that work on the endocrine glands and the sense organs:
   (Headstand - Sirsasana, Inverted Action - Viparita Karani Mudra, and Shoulderstand - Sarvangasana).
5. Those that produce relaxation:
   (Fetal - Garbhasana, Corpse - Savasana, and Crocodile - Makarasana).
6. Those that promote meditation and pranayama:
   (Easy - Sukhasana, Adept - Siddhasana, Lotus - Padmasana, and Thunderbolt - Vajrasana, Hero - Virasana).

Thunderbolt - Vajrasana (Hero - Virasana).

For me, this is an intriguing method of categorization. For these names imply that a change in posture can create a change in attitude and even elicit specific states of consciousness. Yogis have found that when asanas are done properly, they stimulate the quality that they are named for. Hero pose (Virasana) done in the prescribed manner will promote the feeling of courage, self-confidence and stamina. The Lotus pose (Padmasana) will generate an opening of the lotus petals of the subtle body's charkas, producing a feeling of emotional and spiritual expansion. The Adepts pose (Siddhasana) will generate a field of consciousness wherein the practitioner experiences a supreme detachment (Pratyahara) from the sensory world, enabling them to have power over their choices rather than be led by unconscious or previous patterns of behavior. The Thunderbolt pose (Vajrasana), done by a subtle change from Hero pose (Virasana) to stimulate the Vajra nadi in the urethra, brings to realization that there is a wand like column of light (lingam) in the subtle body that extends from the pelvis to the realm of pure consciousness (Siva). Bharadvajasana, a spinal twist, is named for a sage who was one of the seven Rishis of the Rig-Veda. He was responsible for the transmission of Ayurveda from the realms of mythological cosmic intelligences (Indra and the Ashwins) to benefit humanity. By sustained practice of this asana, the student gains access to the plane of consciousness, accessing wisdom (Vijnanamaya kosha). These are not merely statements of Vedic mythology; they are truths accessible to those who apply themselves to follow the path that has been delineated. Why reinvent the wheel?

Asanas can also be classified according to the muscles stretching or strengthened as in my previous book – Structural Yoga Therapy (based on an analysis of postures done with the attention to postural alignment that has become standardized from the teachings of Iyengar Yoga). Yet another perspective is to categorize postures according to the Ayurvedic dosha that they stimulate. David Frawley and Sandra Kozak have categorized Iyengar Yoga style asanas in this manner, although I do not recommend it as it is impractical.[58]

At first perspective, many students seek to simplify the effects the Yoga postures have on the doshas. A common view is that those that push the seat of the dosha, stimulates it. Thus, forward bends are compressing the pelvis making them Vata enhancing and cooling. Spinal twists compress the abdominal region enhancing

Pitta, making their effect heating. Shoulderstand compresses the neck region increasing Kapha, making its benefit cooling. This is a narrow perspective and does not take into consideration a host of other factors that might stimulate the asana to affect the doshas differently. Among the considerations are the complexity of the student's constitution, the manner or length of time in which the posture is held, the mental attention or lack of it, use of breathing and pranayama, the use of bandhas, the time of day and season in which it was done.

According to BKS Iyengar's daughter Geeta, "some asanas have the tendency to stir up heat, hunger, thirst, digestion, and circulation, thus helping to reduce Vata and Kapha. Others have the tendency to create a cooling, soothing, and nourishing sensation. They bring about the condensation of tissues and control excessive secretions in glands and organs. These asanas regulate the Pitta and blood by modifying the intensity of circulation. In addition, the same asana can create heat in one place in the body and cool it in another place. For example, forward extension cools the kidneys, heart, brain, and reproductive and endocrine systems, but heats the digestive system." [59]

The Ayurvedic cycle within a Yoga Pose

"There are three stages in the performance of the asana, namely, assuming the asana (arambha), remaining in the asana (sthiti) and concluding the asana to regain the normal position of the body (visarjan). Each of these three steps has a therapeutic value and psychological effect."[60]

Vata represents initiating motion. It is the first activity of any event. As you first move from where you are into some new position you are increasing Vata. Vata is increased by motion. By moving harmoniously in coordination with your breath to heighten your awareness, Vata will become balanced. As it does, prana will naturally arise and help redirect intuition to a connection with your self that manifests as peace.

Once the motion is underway, the intermediate phase represents Pitta. In this phase, the activity stimulates warmth and circulation. The Pitta phase is going towards a goal; it is increased by desire to change, and the challenge of competition. By cultivating a resolution to purify yourself and keep the fire of your vitality centered in the belly, Pitta becomes balanced. As Pitta becomes balanced, tejas as a spiritual light will arise, directing attention to those activities that produce luminosity and feelings of lightness.

Kapha is the final cycle of activity bringing completion to projects. It is the process of working hard that develops strength, maintaining your commitment to the project that promotes stamina and sustaining it until the activity or motion returns to stillness. Competition reaches its culmination and one becomes satisfied. The stability of Kapha nurtures and feeds. Kapha is increased by stillness. Kapha is balanced by using your strength and stamina towards the subtler level, generating ojas by opening your heart and ultimately finding your own self as the

Divine Presence.

The cycle within asana is a circle. It begins with Vata starting the motion. Pitta going to the pose. Kapha holding the pose. Pitta coming back toward starting position. Vata relaxing and releasing the effects of the pose, thus returning to starting position in an elevated state.

As you come back out of a pose, the last 1/3 of the motion affirms the gain or changes made by the asana. According to how you end the pose, you determine how much tissue memory is retained. When the pose is ended strongly, the body remembers the pose and the changed state is the new reality. In the same manner, as you go into an asana, the first third of the motion opens the tissue layers and the energy gates. At this phase, change is possible. The change is affirmed by how you complete the action. When the body gets the message that you want to change, it listens and makes the change. When the message is simply motion then the body affirms that motion. According to Newton's law of motion, an object will continue to move until acted upon by an outside force. This continuity of action can be applied to make the body and mind still, to reinforce current patterns, or to create a new direction for life.

VIII. The Principles of Vinyasa

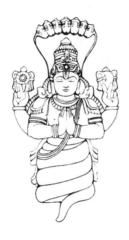

The term Vinyasa means "to proceed step-by-step." The intention is to master a particular asana in a progressive manner by doing variations that lead to the full pose and following its practice, doing counter poses that relieve any potential stress caused by the challenge of the peak asana. It is a logical sequencing of postures following guidelines developed by Professor T. Krishnamacharya (1888 - 1989) that emphasizes a flow of movement that rides on the rhythm of the breath. This unique style is an excellent way to deepen concentration and maximize the effectiveness of Yoga postures.

My first teacher in Krishnamacharya's this method was Paul Copeland, now a child psychiatrist, who taught me in a class situation, unlike Krishnamacharya who taught him in one to one sessions from 1970 until 1972. He was given teaching specific to him and adapted to the fact that he was a young college undergraduate in search of his dharma. When he was in India he was attending musical school learning to play the sitar. The teacher told him he wasn't sitting properly and thus could not hold the instrument in the correct manner to create harmonious chords. He encouraged Paul to do down the street to study Yoga. He was fortunate enough to be one of Krishnamacharya's last students.

The master Yogi encouraged Paul to return to college in America and instead of pursuing music to study physiology in order to research the benefits of Yoga. For this purpose, he gave him training in over fifty specific Vinyasas and ten Pranayamas. He encouraged Paul not to change them, as he claimed they were therapeutic for different conditions. I learned these sequences and over the years discovered that certain sequences were beneficial for the individual Ayurvedic do-shas. Regardless of the Vinyasa, Paul taught me that to round out your practice, relaxation in the Corpse pose, Savasana, should follow each Vinyasa sequence

Through the careful sequencing of Vinyasa form, Yoga poses can be done without the danger of muscle strain in a body unprepared for a specific effort. The sequences are designed to gradually increase in intensity, with the most challenging movements occurring in the second half of the sequence. The muscles and joints are warmed up, worked strongly and safely, and then cooled down once again. Each Vinyasa is an entire routine, equivalent to a brief class.

In 1980, Krishnamacharya's son, TKV Desikachar, taught me the way to design a Vinyasa sequence so that it could be adapted to the individual's needs and present situation. The intensity of the sequence should be gradually increased over the duration of the series. The target pose of the Vinyasa should occur during peak intensity at about two thirds of the period of the entire series. The last third of the time should be spent doing counter poses and gentle variations of the peak asana, since "whatever is done at the end of a series can counteract all that was done before. In fact the same is true with eating and any other activity." [61]

Time of Practice - Intensity

The Yogarahasya composed by the 9th century yogi Nathamuni, strongly influenced Krishnamacharya's teachings. This text gives details on how to adapt to individual needs, recommends Yoga for women, specific asanas for different issues, and the importance of finding a competent teacher. It also describes the benefits of Vinyasa practice:

1. The use of breath to expand/contract
2. Continuous movements produce a concentrated focus of mind
3. The combination of poses in each sequence results in a more balanced "work-out" for the whole body
4. The built-in warm-up/cool-down sequencing ensures a safer, more systematic practice
5. The stamina required to hold a pose comfortably increases gradually
6. Practice is more adaptable to life's changes
7. The poses can be adapted along the spectrum from milder to intense as well as from brief to prolonged.

Vinyasa and Breath

"During the practice of the asanas, one must regulate the inhalation, exhalation and retention of the breath. This depends on the student's capacity.
Slow breathing following the ujjaye technique must be taught." [62]

The practice of Vinyasa quickly shows the importance of proper breathing. In beginning Yoga practitioners, the breath is often shallow (using only the upper half of the chest) and irregular. The flowing movements of Vinyasa encourage the breath to become deeper and more regular, establishing a smooth continuous rhythm in all phases of breathing.

"Without proper practice of the asanas,
it is not possible to master pranayama.
Without the mastery of the prana,
the mind will not be steady." [63]

There is a profound relationship between our mental state, our emotions, and the quality of our breathing. The next time you are sad, angry, or frightened, notice your breath. It is likely to be irregular. Scientific studies have also shown this to be the case. [64] "The quantitative analysis of the respiratory movements for the fundamental cycles showed that for anger, erotic love and tenderness significant changes in amplitude, rate and duration of the 'expiratory pause' were the major elements of differentiation, while for sadness, joy and fear inspiratory over expiratory time ratios were the elements of differentiation." [65]

Vinyasa practice results in the cultivation of a regulated, deep, full breathing pattern that in turn gives a freedom for personal adjustments to become stimulating, sedating, or balancing. Thus, it can easily be utilized for increasing Pitta, Vata, or Kapha. The presentation style may be rajasic, tamasic or sattvic according to the needs of the student.

Practice the ujjaye breath while sitting for approximately three to five minute periods, concentrating on the sound of the breath at the base of the throat. It should not be a nasal sound, but rather a deep throat sound coming from the region near the junction of the collarbones and breastbone. It is necessary to have a qualified teacher check this breath to insure that it is being done properly. This is the ideal type of breathing (pranayama) to use during Vinyasa practice, since it slows the breath and increases concentration. For more details, read the chapter on Pranayama for Vata.

Vinyasa Learning Sequence

In mastering the process of Vinyasa flows, there is a sequence of training that will enable the practice to reach deeply into the experience of Patanjali's guidelines for asana moving into pranayama (YS II, 46-50).

1 - Read through the Vinyasa instructions and check for any potential contra-indi-cated postures. If you identify any, then begin to practice the sequence omit-ting or modifying postures that may be harmful.

2 - Memorize the sequence of motions and breath patterns.

3- When the sequence can be practiced in its entirety uninterrupted, now begin to pay more attention to the breath flow than the postures.

4 - Begin to slow your breathing down so that the sequence will take longer to practice. Vinyasas are done with even ratio (sama vritti) breathing. That is, the inhalation is equal in duration and force to that of the exhalation.

5 – Use Jnana Mudra (thumb and forefinger tip joined) or Yoni Mudra (2 hands forming a down pointing triangle in the space between them) whenever pos-sible.

6 – Deepen the pranayama aspect of the practice by adding pause (kumbhaka) after both the inhalations and exhalations.

7 – During each kumbhaka use mula bandha, releasing it for all breath move-ments.

8 – A final variation is to sandwich the posture between the beginning and end-ing of the breath. In this method, begin inhaling for 3-5 seconds before mov-ing into the first posture. Sustain the inhale for the same 3-5 second interval following the completion of the posture. A similar pattern is maintained during the exhalation phase. This variation creates a profound concentration and is especially beneficial for students who do asana practice prior to their seated meditation practice. The effects will profoundly deepen the ability to enter meditative states more readily.

The Importance of Story Telling

One important aspect of good teaching style is the use of story telling as a way to integrate Yoga practices into a deeper level of the psyche. Yoga is about transformation on all levels and storytelling is a way to allow this to occur, through its ability to reach both sides of the brain.[66]

Swami Muktananda, my spiritual teacher, was adept at story telling, making use of classical stories from his Indian heritage as well as created stories drawn from Sufi and Buddhist traditions.[67]   Swami Prakashananda, my last spiritual mentor, composed stories showing how members of the audience represent archetypes of the story's characters, thus promoting insight into human nature and more specifically into the character of those present.

For each of the Vinyasas I have adapted stories from my teachers and classical sources that will open a door to the inner teachings and awaken you to be able to hear your intuitive guidance more clearly. By hearing the story and reflecting upon its personal or social impact during the practice of the Vinyasas, the sequences can have a more profound affect.

Vinyasas for the Doshas

Vata Vinyasas

The sequences I have chosen for balancing Vata emphasize a deep connection to the breath so that the Prana can be increased and held within your body. These Vinyasas emphasize forward bending motions that are not held for long or with much effort as this tends to imbalance and upwardly displace Vata. They are long sequences challenging concentration and developing the mental strength necessary for contemplation (Dharana) and meditation (Dhyana). With regular practice, they can help the student develop sensitivity to their Prana and over time help to return the five Pranic subdoshas to their home sites.

Vata Vinyasa Sequence
Palm Tree - Balancing Tree - Stick - Auspicious

Pitta Vinyasas

These sequences emphasize opening feelings of spaciousness to the midriff region between the pelvis and the ribcage. While many incorporate backward bending, these poses are meant to be done in an effort that ranges from mild to moderate. When backward bending is overemphasized or done with intensity, it tends to aggravate and upwardly displace Pitta. The pacing for these Pitta Vinyasas is faster than for Vata Vinyasas. Once memorized, the sequences do not need to be done in harmony with the breath, as this element of the practice emphasizes Vata.

Instead the student is focused on the warm sensations to the body of the momentary pauses at the extremes of each motion. The key here is to be able to connect with the energy of enthusiasm and heat, balancing it to purify the physical body. Too much and the body is weakened from the increased rajasic behavior, not enough and one's vitality is not adequate to keep a high level of energy, as tamasic behavior is promoted. When the Pitta Vinyasas are done in this way tejas (the light of spiritual discernment) is developed.

Pitta Dosha Sequence
Cobra - Sunbird - Sun Salutation

Kapha Vinyasas

These sequences promote strength and stamina for the physical body. The poses are challenging for the purpose of developing upper body and cardiovascular strength. Once memorized, they are to be done to challenge your capacity to hold the poses gradually longer. When done repeatedly and slowly, the Vinyasas also can promote an increase in the autoimmune system's function. Inverted poses and variations of the Shoulderstand are particularly instrumental in developing this benefit. Yogis are well known for the ability to remain healthy and are rarely sick because of their capacity to stimulate and balance Kapha. The chest region is especially expanded yet with an underlying softness so that the emotional heart feels open. There is a sense that the shoulders and arms are separated from the chest to become like the wings of the heart. The subtler component is to promote a feeling of ojas as the liquidity of spirit opening your heart to its innate emotions of love and devotion. It does not matter the object of these feelings, but rather that the feelings are expressed and drawn upwards as an offering to the higher power.

Kapha Dosha Sequence
Warrior - Bridge - Shoulderstand

Ayurvedic Vinyasa Sequencing

There are a number of ways that the Vinyasas may be sequenced. They can be practiced in groups according to the dosha that is being balanced, as they are sequenced here. This is the best way to learn this system of Yoga, because it allows you to observe the effects they have upon bringing your subtle elements into harmony. By sequencing in this manner, you can direct attention to uncovering your predominant constitutional quality (Prakruti); balancing Vikruti (the current imbalance), so that you are better able to adapt to the ever changing influences of life.

An advanced method of sequencing appropriate for the student who has regularly practiced these sequences over a year and is familiar with how it influences the doshas through seasonal changes. It places all ten Vinyasas in a longer flowing sequence requiring about an hour of practice (not including other foundational practices such, chanting, and meditation).

Palm Tree - Balancing Tree - Warrior - Bridge - Shoulderstand
Stick - Cobra - Sunbird - Auspicious Pose - Sun Salutation

This sequence will be ideal for those doing pranayama and meditation prior to the Vinyasas so that they can go to work refreshed and invigorated. For those whose lifestyle is free of work schedule and worldly demands, I would recommend doing the Sun Salutation first. Then pranayama and meditation would follow Auspicious Pose Vinyasa to be aligned with the sequence of Patanjali's Classical Ashtanga Yoga Sequence.

IX. Vinyasas for Vata

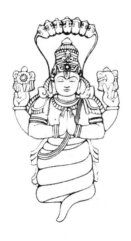

Palm Tree — Tadasana Vinyasa

Tadasana

This is my favorite sequence as it produces a tremendous benefit with a minimum of motions. The sequence lends itself to learning pranayama, mudra, and bandha as they can be applied in ever increasing layers of deepening concentration once the sequence is memorized. It offers a wonderful opportunity to practice the poet Kabir's words –

"Entering into your own body and have a solid place for your feet."

It is a lovely sequence to watch, as it resembles the ideals common also to the Chinese meditation in movement form of Tai Chi Chan, which undoubtedly reached theire from India via Tibet. There are some who believe they may share common roots. Indeed when Krishnamacharya studied with his teacher of seven years, Ram Mohan Brahmachari, they lived in the Lake Manasarovar region of Tibet.

Although Krishnamacharya's student BKS Iyengar calls Tadasana mountain pose, the master rendered tad as a "palm tree" done on the tip toes with arms overhead in an outward fingerlock. [68]

"When the supreme truth is realized, the mind goes away, who knows where; and
who knows how vasana or mental conditioning, karma,
and also joy and despair disappear.
The yogi is then seen to be in a state of continuous and unbroken meditation,
firmly established in adamantine mediation or samadhi, like a mountain." [69]

In contrast, Krishnamacharya rendered tad as a "straight tree"[70] My teacher, Paul Copeland, said that the master's use of English with him was colorful, descriptive, and very full of imagery. He often referred to this "straight tree" as a palm tree moving to the gentle breezes of the ocean. The Palm Tree is a common tree native to the coastal regions of India and the tropics. It is a long slender tree that manages to survive in spite of its sparse root system. In standing position our bodies are like the palm in that we have a small support base relative to our larger upper body. In moving through this Vinyasa, we mimic the gentle swaying motions that this tree makes in response to the wind currents. The Palm Tree is an excellent form in which to learn smoothness in the Vinyasa format of flowing movement and breath symmetry. With practice, the student can learn pacing, conservation of breath, spinal flexibility, and most importantly, concentration.

Krishnamacharya's completed Tadasana posture is a balancing pose done with the arms outstretched overhead, fingers in outward finger lock that draws the abdomen into a mild Uddiyana Bandha, chin down in Jalandhara bandha, feet together with and the heels lifted. The Palm Tree is a common tree native to the coastal regions of India and the tropics. It is a long slender tree that manages to survive in spite of its sparse root system. In standing position our bodies are like the palm in that we have a small support base relative to our larger upper body. In moving through this Vinyasa, we mimic the gentle swaying motions that this tree makes in response to the wind currents. The Palm Tree is an excellent form in which to learn smoothness in the vinyasa format of flowing movement and breath symmetry. With practice, the student can learn pacing, conservation of breath, spinal flexibility, and most importantly, concentration.

The first components of movement free the shoulders, wrists, and upper back. The middle sequence works the mid and lower back as well as hips and inner thighs. The final sequence of movements goes to the extremes of hip, shoulder, and spinal flexion and extension. This sequence is of fundamental importance in preparing you for full forward and backward bending.

Of foremost importance in doing this Vinyasa is to maintain an awareness of breath so that it is continuous throughout the sequence. Only when breath is held is there the likelihood of strain or pain. Breath is the warning sign that can protect us from harm. This sequence is especially beneficial in learning the limits of natural range of motion. Thus it forms the basis of all other standing postures.

The importance of this initial position, Samasthiti "standing stable" with the feet apart, is that it points to the core of our being. It is a path to the central essence of being human. Just standing steady in your own inner being. When in that place, there is another Presence that one begins to notice. That Presence signals that you are never alone. "Sri Bhagavan explained that God means Samasthiti – that is all that is, plus the Be-ing – in the same way as 'Õ' means the individual plus the Being, and the world means the variety plus Be-ing. The Be-ing is in all cases real." [71] This is the central teachings of Yoga as non-dualism. There are very few expressions of this highest level of Yoga. Among them is the story of a sage and his son.

Seed and Tree story Svetaketu & Uddalaka

In the ChhandogyaChandogya Upanishad (part VI, chapter xi, 1-3) is a dialog of the teaching of the sage Uddalaka and his son Svetaketu. "If, my dear, someone were to strike at the root of this large tree it would bleed but live. If he were to strike at the middle, it would bleed but live. If he were to strike at the top, it would bleed but live. Pervaded by the living self, that tree stands firm, drinking in again and again its nourishment and rejoicing. But if the life leaves one of its branches, that branch withers; if it leaves a second, that branch withers, if it leaves a third, that branch withers. If it leaves the whole tree the whole tree withers. In exactly the same manner, my dear, said he, "Know this: This bodies dies, bereft of the living Self, but the living Self dies not. Now, that which is the subtle essence—in it all that exists has its self. That is the Truth. That is the Self. Thou art That, Svetaketu." [72]

"The world is not other than the mind, the mind is not other than the Heart; that is the whole truth." So the Heart comprises all. This is what is taught to Svetaketu by the illustration of the seed of a fig tree.

Contemplation (Dharana) –
"Be strong then, and enter into your own body;
There you have a solid place for your feet.
Think about it carefully!
Don't go off somewhere else!

Kabir says this:
just throw away all thoughts of imaginary things,
and stand firm in that which you are." [73]

Direct your auditory attention to your breath sounds and your visual attention directly in front of you. One exception for visual gaze is during spinal twists in which you will look as far as possible at eye level. The other exception is during backbends when your gaze is upon a spot directly above you.

Precautions –
Anyone with low back pain, sciatica, or in the last trimester of pregnancy should modify the forward bend (steps 11-13) and bend their knees (step 16). If this is still too strenuous (for instance, for those with acute sciatic pain), keep your torso at a 45-degree angle instead of parallel to the floor. Read the instructions carefully before practicing this sequence.

Instructions -
1. Starting position - stand erect with your feet slightly apart and your arms relaxed at your sides. Close your eyes and contemplate the image of a palm tree swaying naturally from the motions of a breeze. Allow your body's natural, gentle rocking motions to occur spontaneously. Contemplate the stillness underlying the motion. This is called Samasthiti, standing steady. Open your eyes and continue to breathe deeply.
2. INHALING as your arms sweep outward and upward while looking up to an upward namaste. EXHALING, look down as you interlace your fingers and turn your palms into an outward finger lock.
3. INHALE as you lift your heels to balance on your toes, coming into Palm Tree Pose (Tadasana). EXHALE, lowering your heels. INHALE and stretch up from your waist with your feet planted.
4. EXHALE, while maintaining the length in your sides, bend to your right. Press your hips to the left while your arms reach to the right.
5. INHALE as you return to the erect centered position.
    EXHALE, bending to your left side. Let your hips move to the right as your

arms move to the left.

INHALE as you return to center.

6. EXHALE, twisting your torso to the right, squeezing your thighs to maintain a straight line from hands to feet. Tilt your head up to look to the back of your hands.

7. INHALE, returning to center, head and eyes level.

EXHALE, twisting to the left, tilt your head upward, stretching your arms outward.

INHALE, returning to center.

8. EXHALE, lower your arms palms down to shoulder height. Then INHALE, rotate the shoulders outward so your palms turn up.

9. EXHALE, twist to the left, gaze at your thumb, while maintaining a straight line across your arms.

INHALE, returning to center position.

EXHALE and twist to the right, looking at your thumb.

10. INHALE, return to center while bringing your hands overhead in an outward finger lock.

11. EXHALE, pressing your pelvis backward to elongate your spine as you come to Half Forward Bend (Ardha Uttanasana).

12. INHALE, open your arms straight out from your shoulders, with your palms down.

13. EXHALE, sweep your palms together aligned to your back in an outward Palm Salute.

14. INHALE initiate an upward movement from your hands returning to standing with your arms overhead shoulder width apart.

15. EXHALE, reaching forward from your chest as you extend your hips backward into a full forward bend. Place your fingertips along the line of your toes, bending your knees if necessary. INHALE, stretching your head and chest forward elongating your spine.

16. EXHALE lower your head toward your shins and press your palms toward the floor coming to a full forward bend (Uttanasana). While keeping fingertips fixed to the floor, repeat inhaling up and exhaling downward twice more, progressively bringing your forehead closer to your shins.

17. INHALE reaching outward to pull yourself up, returning to erect standing arms overhead.

18. EXHALE spreading your arms outward and behind your back then interlace your fingers while pulling your shoulders back to expand your chest. This is Karmasana, pose of karma.

19. INHALE squeeze your shoulders and go into a lifted backbend looking overhead.

20. EXHALE bending forward while pulling your arms away from your back. An option is to stay in the pose for three full breaths, while allowing gravity to deepen your stretch.

21. INHALE returning to standing erect.
22. EXHALE round your shoulders forward to bring your palms together behind your back into a reverse Namaste.
23. INHALE pulling your shoulders together to flatten your hands, expand your chest to look upward.
24. EXHALE twisting to the left, squeezing your shoulder blades, while bringing your head level.
    INHALE returning to center.
    EXHALE reverse twist to the right side.
    INHALE returning to center.
25. EXHALE lifting your chest and firm your buttocks as you backbend and look upward.
    INHALE returning to center.
26. EXHALE coming into a gentle forward bend dropping your head.
27. INHALE return to center standing position.
    EXHALE lower your arms to sides, while stretching out your fingers.
    INHALE bring your palms to Namaste gesture at your heart. Stand in a comfortable, stable position and observe the benefits of the sequence. Take six full breaths, and then lie down to rest for one to two minutes in Savasana.

Notes to polish your practice –

Concentrate on developing this Vinyasa gradually by first memorizing the sequence. It is suggested that you memorize it in segments until the entire sequence can become a flow. The next step is to deepen your pranayama extending the length of the breath with every motion. I recommend that you break down the series learning a few lines at a time. You may want to learn only half the series, ending at pose 14 instead of the entire series. Once you can repeat half the series from memory then you can continue to learn the remainder of the Vinyasa.

Two poses are notably challenging. The first, #15, may be best learned with knees bent until your hip flexors are strong enough to fully extend your spinal columns length. Do not attempt to straighten your knees until the following position can be done with your palms flat upon the floor beside your feet.

The other posture that is awkward is reverse Namaste. As an aid in reversing your hands, round your upper back and turn your elbows forward as you rotate your wrists from fingers down to fingers up position. If your hands will not reverse then an option is to grasp your forearms behind your back with your hands gradually moving closer to your elbows. This will help to keep your chest expanded and develop your upper back strength.

Benefits –

This Vinyasa is a beautiful and graceful sequence composed by Krishnamacharya for Paul Copeland, MD to do research on the physiological benefits of Yoga practices. I find its practice continuing to deepen as I have persisted with it for 30 years. It is simple yet elegant; when done repeatedly with breath symmetry, it balances Vata dosha, promoting regularity of breath and a calm mind.

Many Vata conditions benefit from this practice. Some include CFIDS - chronic fatigue immune dysfunction syndrome, body aches, joint pain, and even chronic conditions of the skeletal system like arthritis and ankylosing spondylitis (a condition in which the bones fuse sometimes with scoliosis and/or kyphosis or hunchback).

There is a story about the fourth century Coptic Christian monk, Apa Bane, founder of one of the first Christian desert monasteries south of Cairo, Egypt. His name means "Father Palm Tree." "Possibly the saint received this epithet after entering the monastery because of his kyphotic appearance which reminded them of a palm tree resisting a desert storm. He lived as an ascetic, ate only in a standing position in his dark cell and slept leaning with his chest supported by a wall erected for this purpose. Perhaps he had difficulty in rising after sitting or lying, and therefore adopted the habit of eating and sleeping in a standing position. In any case, we can assume that the saint did not recognize his stiffness as a disease but assumed it was a fate put upon him by God, which contributed to his unique way of asceticism." [74]   The skeleton of persons with this condition does indeed resemble the lines of growth of the Palm Tree.

When done first thing in the morning, it is a gentle way to warm up the spine and prepare for more difficult practices. With practice you can learn to decompress every segment of the spinal column with this sequence. The movements are coupled with lateral flexion, rotation and hip flexion, which can promote increased circulation to the spinal discs. It is an ideal sequence for adolescents as it can facilitate an erect posture and optimize height. The practice increases the posture of self-esteem. Who can say which comes first, the posture or the esteem? It also lessens the tendencies for mild scoliosis curvatures to become greater during developmental years.

It can stand alone and be a wonderful way to harmonize breath and motion. I particularly enjoy doing it for 3 or up to 10 repetitions as a way of deepening my breath and beginning to connect to the primal field of the Life Force that Uddalaka speaks of. When done for more repetitions, one can begin to deepen and lengthen the pranayama and add steadiness of eye gaze, dristi.

Palm Tree Vinyasa
Tadasana
Mukunda Stiles ©2006

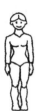 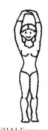 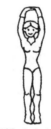 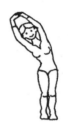 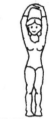

1- Steady Pose
Samasthiti

2- INHALE upward
salute. EXHALE-
outward fingerlock

3- INHALE raise heels
balancing in Palm Tree
Pose. EXHALE, heels down
INHALE, stretch up

4- EXHALE side
bend

5- INHALE center
repeat 4-5 other
side.

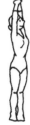 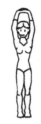 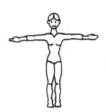 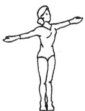 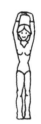

6- EXHALE twist &
look up.

7- INHALE center
Reverse twist.

8- EXHALE lower arms
INHALE turn palms up

9- EXHALE twist
look at thumb
Reverse twist.

10- INHALE lace
fingers outward
fingerlock

   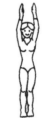 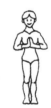

11- EXHALE half
forward bend

12- INHALE spread
arms across

13- EXHALE arms
forward in Namaste.

14- INHALE erect

15- EXHALE center
with Namaste.
OPTION is end here

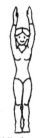

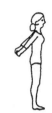

15- EXHALE palms to floor
beside feet. INHALE, arch
back, head up.

16- EXHALE head to legs
in Intensive Stretch Pose -
Uttanasana. Repeat 15-16
three times.

17- INHALE raise up arms
over head

18- EXHALE interlace
fingers behind back
Pose of Karma -
Karmasana

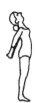

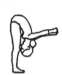

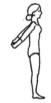

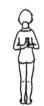

19- INHALE squeeze
shoulders, look up.

20- EXHALE forward
bend pulling arms away
from back.

21- INHALE return to
erect posture.

22- EXHALE reverse
Namaste or hold elbows,
back is rounded.

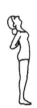

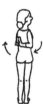

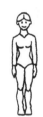

23- INHALE head up
squeeze shoulders

24- EXHALE head level
as you turn right
INHALE, center
EXHALE, to left
INHALE, center

25- EXHALE lift chest
hips firm back bend
looking up.
INHALE center.

26- EXHALE gentle
forward bend.

27- INHALE center
EXHALE lower arms
return to center.

Balancing Tree — Vrksasana Vinyasa

Vrksasana

This sequence is named for the Balancing Tree pose (Vrksasana). It is also known as Bhagirathasana, named for the sage whose devotional sincerity to Shiva resulted in the heavenly river Ganga being manifested on Earth. This posture promotes a feeling of equanimity and serenity. Its practice is described in the medieval Tantra Hatha text the <u>Gheranda Samhita</u> in chapter II, sutra 36.

The qualities of a tree are used in several places in yogic teachings. Patanjali's eightfold path is more literally rendered as "eight limbs;" symbolically a tree with eight limbs, that must each be cultivated for the fulfillment of the promised experiences he describes leading to illumination.

By the sustained practice of all the component limbs of Yoga,
the impurities dwindle away and wisdom's radiant light shines forth. [75]

A tree's image is used metaphorically as the fullness, the continuity of human experience. By denying any of the states of life, the life force is diminished and fulfillment is lost.

"What are seen as birth, death, pain, pleasure, form and formlessness are all limbs of one being. There is no division among them, even as there is no division in the several parts of one tree." [76]

Another balancing pose of this Vinyasa is the Dancer King posture (Natarajasana) which symbolizes Shiva as witness consciousness. It is named after Nataraja, the Cosmic Lord or the Lord of the Dance of time. The Dancer King is the subject of a statue of Shiva dancing on the back of a dwarf, where Shiva symbolizes the ignorance of our True Self. By focusing on the witness consciousness, one can learn to transcend human frailties and difficulties with equanimity, while remaining fully engaged in the daily routine of everyday life.

Contemplation (Dharana) –
A regular practice of balancing postures can enhance our humility. It is natural that we will fall. No one can maintain balance forever, so it is important to learn how to fall with grace and even with a sense of laughter and playfulness.

During a mid-life crisis I nurtured myself by taking time away from teaching yoga to live amongst the redwood forests of Northern California. While there, an empathic Yoga teacher nurtured me back to spiritual health by numerous acts of kindness. On one of our many walks together in the forest, he showed me an enormous redwood tree that had fallen during a winter storm about two years prior. The tree's root ball was remarkably shallow being only about three feet deep yet it was easily 50' in diameter. The trunk was nearly 30' in diameter, the length of the tree having shattered into five major sections upon impact when it fell and its 270'length (its former height) was gracing the fern-covered forest floor. Its age was estimated to be over 2000 years. I was awe struck! How remarkable is the strength of this majestic being and how awesome its return to earth. The circle of life was never revealed to me as complete as in the presence of this being, whose relatives are the largest living beings.

The Story of Queen Julia [77]

Queen Julia loved her subjects so much that she was constantly attending to their affairs and seeking to uplift the quality of their lives. She was so busy with their lives that she rarely had time for herself. Inevitably, yet quite predictably, this lifestyle created a profound sickness due to increasing stress. She was forced to go into solitude to recover. Her attendant recommended she go to visit the summer palace that her predecessor had built in the milder climate prevalent in the south of the country. The journey was a delight for the countryside was truly exquisite. Seeing such abundance of nature's greenery, Julia remarked how much she felt nourished simply by being immersed in the colors and aromas of nature. During her journey, Queen Julia heard of a famous woman saint named Mira who was said to be "wise beyond measure." The Queen decided to seek her out for counsel as to how she might better serve her subjects and herself simultaneously.

Upon their meeting Mira saw deeply into the burden Queen Julia was carrying. Mira invited Queen Julia to go for a walk in the forest to greet her subjects. Mira explained to the Queen that all of nature was her domain, and that the love and empathy of every tree and plant were with her constantly.   As they walked on suddenly Mira grabbed the trunk of one of the greatest trees Queen Julia had ever seen. At first Mira seemed entranced as an exquisite glow radiated from her and her smile turned into a saintly expression of love. Then she began to scream, "The tree has got me and won't let me go!"

Queen Julia was shocked, "How can a tree grab and hold you? Have you gone mad?"

Mira replied with a look of delight, "How then can your subjects hold onto you? Can you not cast them off as easily as I relax my grip on this magnificent tree?" Saying so she released her embrace of the tree and she fell upon the lush forest floor laughing hysterically. The Queen's illness faded away soon after due to her sharing in the lifestyle and loving company of the saintly Mira.

Precautions -

While none of the poses are strenuous or harmful, they are challenging to your sense of equilibrium. If this is a concern then you might want to do the series close to a wall or chair in case you want more reliable support.

Instructions -

1. Start by standing in Samasthiti pose with your feet hips width and hands at your sides. Take several deep breaths, centering your attention and focusing

on enhancing your sense of poise. Continue standing until you notice a natural tendency to sway and your body's tendency to make continuous adjustments as it maintains center. Then gently extend yourself taller, lengthening through your spine, neck, and skull. Experience how a tree would reach to the warmth and radiance of the sunlight.

2. On an INHALE, bring your palms together into Namaste (Palm Salute gesture) at your heart. Continue to elongate your spine while taking three comfortable breaths. To steady your balance, gaze at a fixed point and feel the solidity of the earth.

3. EXHALE and bending your right knee bring it straight forward as high as possible, then externally rotate your hip without twisting your pelvis to rest your foot on your inner thigh. Remain steady for three breaths, then on an

4. INHALE extend your arms straight up overhead, keeping palms together in Namaste. Stay steady for three breaths.

5. EXHALE as you lower your arms to your sides, returning your leg to the ground.
    REPEAT steps 2 - 5 with your left leg lifted.

6. EXHALE lowering your hands to bring your right foot into the upper groin with your knee to the side. Place your heel on the thick gracilis tendon that attaches to your pubic bone.

7. INHALE drawing your hands up to Namaste at your heart and extend through the posture steadying your balance for three breaths. Then on an

8. INHALE extend your arms straight up. Hold the Balancing Tree pose (Vrksasana) for three breaths, maintaining your balance by keeping your inner and outer thighs firm. Then on an

9. EXHALE sweep your hands out and down, simultaneously bringing your knee forward then downward returning to Standing Steady pose.
    REPEAT (6 - 9), balancing on your right leg.

10. INHALE extending your spine and chest to full capacity then as you EXHALE bend your right knee bringing your foot behind your hip, grasp the top of your ankle with your right hand.

11. INHALE extend your left arm forward and upward, gently pulling your arms away from each other. Steady your balance for three breaths.

12. INHALE lift your chest fully lengthening your spine as your pull your foot away from your hips coming into the Dancer pose (Natarajasana). Equalize the pull of your foot backward to the expansion of your chest forward.

13. INHALE comes to standing erect with your knees together, heel pulled toward your hip, while lifting your left arm straight up.

14. EXHALE using both hands pull your heel firmly toward your buttocks with thighs together.

15. INHALE while opening your chest, then EXHALE and release your leg returning to Standing Steady position.
    REPEAT (10 - 15), balancing on your right leg, with your left leg lifted.

16. INHALE as you bring your arms overhead, with your palms facing each other.
17. EXHALE lowering your hips into a partial squat position squeezing your thighs together.
18. INHALE lengthening your spine then EXHALE into a deeper squat, then INHALE bringing yourself into a vertical line.
19. EXHALE as you balance on your toes with your thighs parallel to the floor. INHALE sitting tall then hold the pose steadily for three breaths.
20. INHALE forming Namaste to your heart bringing yourself into the full Squat pose, Utkatasana. EXHALE fully then as you
21. INHALE come to be standing as you extend your arms overhead.
22. EXHALE as you bring your hands to your heart in Namaste to finish the Vinyasa. Take several deep, full breaths while feeling the benefits of the series.

Notes to polish your practice -

The eyes are very important for maintaining balance. Fixed gaze (Tratak), described in chapter five on Yoga Purification Practices, is to be maintained without an attempt to see details in the objects you are observing. Maintain a relaxed gaze. By fixing your gaze on an unmoving object, the process of concentration begins automatically. Your breath will become smooth, regular, and slow. There may be a tendency to hold your breath, yet by staying alert, the rhythm will establish itself.

Work to keep your hips and pelvis level and square to the front throughout the Vinyasa. This will allow the muscles of your inner and outer thighs to adapt to changing pressures of gravity and maintain a balanced posture. Feel the stability of the pose not only at your foot and ankle, but also in the firm position of your pelvic girdle.

Many people have a tendency to do the Balancing Tree posture with their bent thigh straight out to the side. Since normal range of motion of the hips in abduction is only 45°, this 90° motion is impossible without twisting your pelvis. This places the hips uneven from side to side and gives a twist in the spinal column.

Benefits -

The Balancing Tree builds on the Palm Tree sequence. While the Palm Tree develops rhythm in breath and motion, the Balancing Tree develops concentration and poise. Because it requires us to focus our mind and stay with our breath while poised on one leg, this sequence deepens our inner work. Balancing poses are said to impart stability and greater self-esteem.

Physical balance can lead to a stronger, more determined mental and psychological stance. The quality of maintaining your balance in life without strain or wavering can be enhanced through the practice of this Vinyasa. You will notice that when you are having trying times in life, the balancing poses are likely to be more difficult. However, practice during these times often makes the difficulties of life seem less stressful as it may promote insights into those situations.

Because the arm positions in the Vinyasa lift your chest and diaphragm, enabling the diaphragm to move more powerfully, the sequence is ideal for anyone with respiratory limitations or shallow breathing patterns that often accompany depression.

The variations of hip height in squatting are excellent for strained ligaments of the knee, though if your knee strain is obvious, be sure to keep your feet a more comfortable distance apart. Usually increasing your width from six to twelve inches apart will promote comfort while increasing stamina. The Squat pose also enhances the opening and strengthening of the diaphragm, bringing vitality into breathing. It requires a lift of the rib cage and separates the ribs fully. In the full squat position, the ankles are stretched intensively, and so balance may be precarious. If there is a balancing problem, move your feet even wider apart. Keep the inner arch of your foot lifted to help support your ankle.

Utkatasana, or the Squat pose, resembles the position of a chair in the half version (position 22). The full version is done by balancing on the tiptoes, so it is very awkward and is sometimes called "the hazardous pose" or "the uneven pose." Utkatasana is mentioned in the <u>Gheranda Samhita</u> in Chapter 2, Sutra 23, with just a brief description. The Squat posture tones the adductor muscles of the inner thigh. In addition, the bending of the knees strengthens the quadriceps muscles that stabilize and straighten knee joints.

Many of the benefits of Yoga we can only speculate at, since it is nearly impossible to do an accurate physiological study of its benefits. For instance, attempts at balance will develop our capacity to adapt thus certainly strengthening our immune system, the master adapter.   But how much this may benefit us is probably impossible to measure. We can feel the results of Yoga as the "improved sense of well being," more than that I shall leave to the Yoga scientists to uncover. They have discovered many of the mysterious ways in which Yoga could or has benefited our various physiological systems.

Practice of the Balancing Tree Vinyasa strengthens the joints of the legs and hips and removes strains caused by over-exertion or exercise done with improper alignment. This is an ideal sequence to practice before running or swimming. It tends to balance Vata dosha while sedating an over active Pitta dosha.

Balancing Tree Vinyasa
Vrksasana
Mukunda Stiles © 1991

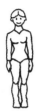
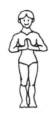
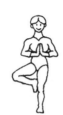
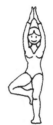
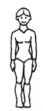

1- INHALE in
Mountain Pose
Tadasana

2- INHALE palms to
Namaste

3- EXHALE right foot
to left inner thigh

4- INHALE hands
to up namaste
Tree Pose - Vrksasana

5- EXHALE lower
hands & leg.
Reverse side, 2-5

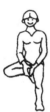
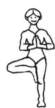
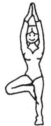
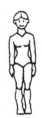

6- EXHALE right heel
to upper groin.

7- INHALE palms to
namaste. EXHALE then

8- INHALE arms up
in Namaste

9- EXHALE lower hands
& leg. Reverse side, 6-9.
INHALE then

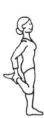
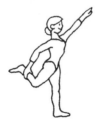
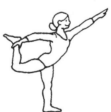
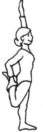
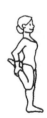

10- EXHALE right
heel to hip

11- INHALE left arm up
EXHALE then

12- INHALE extend chest, lift
knee. EXHALE- Dancer King
Natarajasana

13- INHALE, erect
heel to hip.

14- EXHALE both
hands pull heel
to hip.

Stick — Dandasana Vinyasa

Dandasana

The name of this series comes from a reference to Meru Danda, which is a Tantrik term for the spinal column. In Tantrik Yoga, a central principle concept is that which is outside is also inside. According to Hindu mythology, there is a golden mountain, known as Mount Meru, in the causal plane of the Himalayas that is the axis of the universe. Upon that mountain is a heavenly residence for all the deities, known as Shambhala. When the mind is focused due to a strong will and the discipline of consistent meditation, the energy centers become charged and transform the spine that connects the centers. Then a mystical staff (or stick) is created, capable of revealing hidden supernatural abilities. They are the deities within each individual. The power source that activates healing energies then materializes. The caduceus, the medical emblem, is the Western symbol of these latent healing powers.

Contemplation (Dharana) -

Sit in Stick posture with your legs extended and hands behind your hips with fingers pointing backward. Then adjust the placement of your arms so that you can begin to feel evenness to both your back and your arms. To facilitate this, lift your chest and keep your legs firmly together. Next begin to relax the effort of your arms until you feel the full length of your spinal column being lengthened. Hold your eyes steady, either closed or open to deepen your concentration. Adjust yourself to feel your spine not simply your back. Stay with this awareness continuously. Do not waver but make a resolution in your mind to remain steady with a comfortable yet sustained effort to elongate your spinal column.

Continue to adjust your pose until the effects generate the process of selective relaxation. Your goal is to empower your spinal column and then to release the layers of body that hide the subtle Stick and its energy centers from your perspective. Exert an upward pull yet relax the effort until you can uncover the naturally arising Udana Prana opening your chest and head. It will slowly become more distinct as your body releases its hold on your mind. Your energy body will awaken as you detach the effort from your musculature. By persistence you will uncover your chakras and the naturally arising force that nurtures your evolution from matter to Spirit. Stay still for at least 10 minutes.

Meru Danda and the Unfolding of the Chakras

The Meru Danda spoken of at the beginning of Dandasana Vinyasa notes is within us as the central canal. This place is also referred to as the central most essence of our continually evolving body.

At the base of the Mountain that is our body is the primal energy center known as Muladhara Chakra. This "root" chakra is composed of the earth element. With it comes the psychological qualities we associate with feelings of security, stability and groundedness. As the spiritual dimensions open they reveal a connection to the creative forces personified as Brahma and Sarasvati. These forces stabilize us through their expressions in art, dance, literature, and the process of learning.

Just above this center is the second chakra, the Svadhisthana. Its location is at the top of the pubic region for men and at the cervix for women. It is composed of the elemental qualities of water expressed as fluidity, openness, sensuality, and pleasure. This energy center is often sensed as feminine and its name translates as "in Her own abode." Goddess Shakti is most at home here. Vishnu and Lakshmi play here, generating feelings of abundance and prosperity. The energies available to us from this chakra give sensual and sexual pleasure.

The third chakra or Manipura is composed of the qualities of the element fire. It is a place of passion from which we generate the fulfillment of dharma. Located in the region of the navel, the name means "filled with gems," implying a source of abundant wealth. It is sometimes confused with the solar plexus (a physical nerve center) located well above the navel. Through the activities of right livelihood and selfless service to others, our fire expresses itself in the most wholesome manner. When this energy becomes confused with the previous chakra, stress will result. However, our duty to others is not to be a source of pleasure, merely a place to learn selflessness. Only when this is done can we be truly stress free and generate the uplifting qualities that promote an awakening of the next chakra. The qualities of Shiva as stability, stillness, and empowerment manifest as being at home with your role in the world. In contrast, the qualities of Kali as Shiva's consort are also found here. She is the discriminator between righteous actions and inappropriate actions.

The fourth chakra or Anahata ("unstruck sound") represents the air element. Its home is at the center of the chest. It represents a sense of openness and possibility. As the heart opens, it produces a sense of higher consciousness. This center is the transition place marking the distinction from Hatha to Raja Yoga. There is no form here as the Spirit of guidance transcends personification, generating a sound that is naturally arising without any form to strike it into existence. Thus it preexists all forms, being of the element air.

The fifth chakra or Vishuddhi ("purification" center) has no true form as it is the manifestation of the element ether. It has a sense of spaciousness and vastness. We cannot see it; we can only expand ourselves to its vastness. There is clarity of communication as the voice reaches a primal resonance manifesting what might be called the consciousness of a sage. Though it has no deity representing it, all the chakras below this have form.

The sixth chakra is the third eye or Ajna chakra and is beyond the elements. It is pure intuition and guidance. The word Ajna means "command," implying that only when Spirit gives the command can one truly transcend the physical domain. The mind can perceive above the chakra but what it perceives is itself. To truly go beyond the chakra means to go beyond thought and for that, a secret door must

be opened. The presence of the guru or inner teacher must command that the veil
be lifted and inner sight given to pass beyond the mists of the mind.

The final chakra is the crown or Sahasrar, the "thousand petaled" center. It
covers the full range of the mind as consciousness yet is above the mind, generating spiritual insights that transcend what was previously accessible. This place is
entered through samadhi, absorption into the essence of Spirit.

Precautions –

A person with low back weakness should be cautious during all forward bending movements. It is better to work with a mild stretch in the back and hamstrings,
gradually lengthening the time spent in the pose. The ideal is to feel the posture
evenly in your back and legs. For sciatica, bend your knees during all forward
bends to lessen the stretch to the nerve. This is not therapy for sciatica but will
lessen the tendency for inflammation to the nerve.

Instructions -

1.   Begin by sitting in Stick pose. Externally rotate your shoulders to open your
     chest and aid in lifting your back. Keep your head level and gaze directed
     forward.
2.   INHALE and swing your arms out to the sides, joining them in an overhead
     Namaste gesture.
     Then EXHALE into an outward finger lock. Stay in this position for a total
     of three breaths continuing to extend your back and legs while keeping your
     arms beside your ears.
3.   EXHALE lowering your arms to starting position while supporting your open
     chest.
4.   INHALE raise your arms forward sweeping them overhead with palms facing
     each other.
5.   EXHALE and slowly tilt your pelvis backward curling your spine to the floor.
     Extend your arms palms upward overhead on the floor. Stretch from hands
     to feet for three breaths.
6.   EXHALE sitting up to take hold of your legs. INHALE contracting your hip
     flexors to lengthen your back.
7.   EXHALE, move your torso forward leading with your chest, allow your head
     to hang in between your arms. REPEAT 6 and 7 three times progressively
     bringing your abdomen up over your legs and chest. This posture is the
     Westside Back Stretch pose - Paschimottanasana.
8.   On the fourth INHALE extend your arms fully outward then upward to sit
     erect.
9.   EXHALE return to Stick pose, lowering your arms and placing your hands a
     foot behind your hips.
10. INHALE, lifting your chest then pelvis, keeping your knees firm forming
     a straight line from your feet to your head. This is Eastside Front Stretch,

Purvottanasana.

11. EXHALE lower your hips by bending your knees and separating your feet hip width.

12. INHALE lift your chest then your hips, forming a straight line from knees to shoulders. This is Table pose, Chatuspadapitham, literally the Four Limbs Supported pose.

13. EXHALE and lower your hips returning to position 11.

14. INHALE bringing your arms forward parallel to the floor; slowly straighten your legs to in the Boat pose, Navasana. Take three breaths.

15. EXHALE by pelvic tilting your waist backward, slowly roll your spine to the floor, going into Relaxation pose, Savasana, with your legs apart and palms up at your sides. Adjust your posture so you can fully relax and remain for 5 minute.

Notes to polish your practice –

The Stick pose, though simple to picture, is difficult to master because in order to support the spine it requires strength in your hip flexors, located at the upper front of your thighs. Signs of weakness in these muscles are common; they include a rounding of the lower back and thus an inability to sit upright without the aid of your arms. In this case it is better to place your hands farther and wider away from your hips so that your latissimus dorsi muscle can assist in developing stamina in your hip flexors. For those whose back is strong, the pose can be done with little or no weight upon your palms.

I recommend doing this posture with the fingers pointing backward as this protects the wrists from overstretching. Some Yoga teachers insist on having the fingers forward and this hyperflexes the wrist. As normal range of motion of the wrist is 80° (less than a right angle), I find this can strain or even cause carpal tunnel syndrome. This is particularly an issue for students who are subject to repetitive motion syndrome of keyboarding. Reversing the fingers keeps wrist flexion to a safer angle. An even more conservative position would be to place the hands farther back from the hips.

Westside Back Stretch pose from a lying position minimizes the strain to the lower back by allowing a progressive sequence of movements into the completed posture. Working with the breath to extend the spine then flex it encourages a contrast of strengthening, relaxing, and stretching that works progressively through the full range of motion of the spinal column. For persons with pain in the legs or back regardless of its source, it is safer to bend the knees in phase six. If the pain does not return then they can slowly straighten the knees during position seven.

Eastside Front Stretch is the counterpose to the Westside Back Stretch. Together, these poses create a beautiful balance in strengthening the back as well as giving it flexibility. The Eastside Front Stretch especially develops strength in the posterior shoulder compartment comprised of the posterior deltoid, latissimus dorsi and the triceps brachii. It also strengthens the hip extensor muscles, composed of the hamstrings and the gluteus maximus. It is safest when the upper body lift is done first. Lifting in reverse sequence - from the hips with shoulders following -may strain your lumbar region.

Table pose (Chatuspadapitham) utilizes similar muscles to the previous pose, except that bending the knees to a right angle increases the challenge to the hip extensors. The hamstrings are not used as efficiently as in previous postures, so it requires more strength of the gluteal muscles to maintain hip extension and keep the pelvis level to the shoulder and knee height. The principle muscle responsible for Boat pose (Navasana) is the psoas, the deepest hip flexor, in combination with your abdominals. The perfection of the "V" shape of the pose comes from a balance of strength of the hip flexors (especially the psoas) with their antagonist the rectus abdominis and synergists, the erector spinae. Together, these muscle groups keep the back erect. The Boat pose creates strength and heat in the abdominal area, and if practiced frequently can help to maintain the "gastric fire" - the ability to digest food efficiently.

Dandasana, the Stick posture, is mentioned in the oldest existent commentary on Patanjali's Yoga Sutras II, 46, which describes the practice of asana. This commentary by the sage Vyasa was written in the 6th century AD. In his commentary, he lists, without further description, nine postures as examples that can help the body to become steady and comfortable in preparation for pranayama and meditation practices.

Benefits –
The Stick Vinyasa strengthens your back and stimulates the spinal nerves. Its benefits extend to both your gross and subtle physical body. It can influence the subtle energy body when your mind is focused through holding the Stick Pose and the Westside Back Stretch for greater durations. The subtle body is also stimulated by maintaining the rhythm and evenness of the breath. These practices add depth to your concentration during Vinyasa and also prolong the naturally arising experiences of meditation.

> *"Paschimottanasana, the foremost of all asanas,*
> *causes the prana to flow through the back, strengthens digestion,*
> *reduces weight, and bestows health."*
> Hathayoga PradipikaI, 29

Paschimottanasana is also mentioned in two other Tantrik Hatha texts, the Shiva-Samhita (Chapter 3, sutras 108-112) and the Gheranda-Samhita (Chapter 2, sutra 26). The Shiva Samhita III, 108-112, calls it Ugrasana, which means "powerful or formidable pose," claiming that it removes lethargy and sluggishness from the body and that it excites the motion of Prana, and thus creates spiritual heat or tapas, to burn our attachment to sensual desires. A balance must be struck so that our craving for sensuality (kama) does not overpower our desire for self realization (moksha).

"Bondage is the craving for pleasure, and its abandonment is liberation." [78]

Stick Vinyasa
Dandasana
Mukunda Stiles © 2007

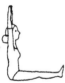

1- Stick Pose, place hands to extend back.

2- INHALE, raise arms upward Salute. EXHALE outward fingerlock. Take 3 breaths

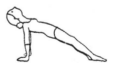

3- EXHALE, palms back of hips, take 3 breaths.

4- INHALE, arms up palms face each other

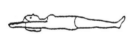

5- EXHALE lay down keeping legs together. Extend the spine for 3 breaths. INHALE fully then

6- EXHALE, forward bend, hold legs. INHALE raise chest to extend your back.

7- EXHALE, move forward to Westside Back Stretch Paschimottanasana Repeat 6-7, 3 times.

8- INHALE, arms up palms face each other.

9- EXHALE, palms on floor 12" behind hips.

10- INHALE, raise body in one line, legs together, Eastside Front Stretch Purvottanasana.

11- EXHALE lower hips knees bent, feet hip width apart.

12- INHALE, lift hips in line with knees. Table Pose - Chatuspadapitham '4 leg support'

13- EXHALE, hips down.

14- INHALE, hold legs straight. Boat Pose - Navasana

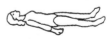

15- EXHALE, relax to floor, legs and arms apart. Corpse Pose - Savasana

Auspicious — Bhadrasana Vinyasa

Bhadrasana

Vyasa is the earliest author to use the name Bhadrasana in his commentary on Patanjali's Yoga Sutras dated to the 6th century CE. It is also cited in three other classical Tantrik Hatha texts - the Hatha Yoga Pradipika (I, 53-43); the Vasistha Samhita (I, 77) and the Gheranda Samhita (II, 9-10). Most contemporary students of Yoga know the pose as the Bound Angle pose, Baddha Konasana. In this pose the student's body resembles a pyramid with the base corners being the pelvis, knees and the soles of the feet. This is a posture of integrity, one that gives a sense of auspiciousness in just being human. We are unique in all the species; we have self-awareness and through that quality we can come to know the hidden or True Self.

The Body as a Pyramid

Contemplation (Dharana) –

As you sit in this posture with a meditative state, shift your attention to your energy body and the vital points (marmas) that connect it to your physical body. At the center of every joint in your body is a minor chakra, a power point of the energy grid that connects the five dimensional states (koshas) of body/emotions/mind/intuition/Spirit into a sense of wholeness.

Begin by lightly touching the major energy points located at your inner knees, followed by the chakras located at your perineum (between the anus and genitals), pubic bone, navel, center of your chest, center of your forehead (3rd eye), and crown of your head. In your mind's eye begin to connect the energy of your knee chakras to your navel. Repeat this several times. By touching these points you can stimulate the flow of Samana Prana. Once this prana is active you will experience either peristalsis of the digestive organs or a subtle sense of movement circulating outward from your navel. Once a reaction is noted, connect the knee points to the heart center stimulating the upward flow of Udana Prana. Remain for some time until you sense the energy moving unaided by your mind searching for an experience. When you experience a spontaneous upward flow that is the sign that Udana Prana is awakened.

After some time, allow your knee points to connect to an apex located at your third eye. Allow yourself to follow the inner energy guided by intuition. Then feel the overlap of the three upward pointing triangles as you bring attention to all three simultaneously. Practice the art of surrendering to the vitality and creativity of your own Life Force. The word Prana means "that which is present everywhere, at all times." See how this correlates or contrasts with your direct experience. It is important to remember that the subtle body cannot be known by your mind, but by a subtler sense organ we call intuition.

Precautions –

Do not do this sequence if you have severe lower back conditions such as slipped lumbar disc or acute sciatica. Also the student is cautioned to watch for any adverse reactions to their knees. Any pain or discomfort to the medial knee between the kneecap and the posterior tendons of the hamstrings, gracilis and sartorius muscles is to be totally avoided.

Instructions –

1. Start by sitting in the Stick pose so that your back is erect. Take a series of deep full breaths focusing your attention upon lengthening your spinal column.

2. EXHALE as you bring your feet in so that the soles of your feet are together with your knees spread open forming the Auspicious pose, Bhadrasana. Straighten your arms placing the back of your hands on your knees with the tip of your thumbs against the tip of your forefingers. This hand position is Jnana Mudra, the Seal of Wisdom.

3. INHALE as you bring your arms up over your head to Upward Salute, Urdhva Namaste.
   EXHALE as you interlace your fingers turning the palms up to form an outward finger lock.
   INHALE as you extend your spinal column. Stay in this position for three rhythmic breaths.

4. EXHALE as you bend forward while lowering your head, bringing your thumbs to the floor in front of your feet. Encourage the opening of your groin muscles, the adductors, as you pull your knees downward with the tone of your outer hip muscles, your abductors.

5. INHALE as you return to the previous position. Then repeat steps 4 and 5 three times gently encouraging a release in your hips and groin.

6. EXHALE as you lower your hands to catch hold of your ankles. INHALE extend your spine to sit tall.

7. EXHALE and as you bend forward, bring your elbows onto your lower inner thighs. INHALE lengthen upward then EXHALE as you press out and down from your shoulders to open your groin, bringing your knees closer to the floor. Repeat steps 6-7 three times.

8. INHALE and sit up with your palms together overhead in Upward Salute.

9. EXHALE bring your hands to the floor, fingers backward well behind your hips. INHALE as you lift your chest. EXHALE as you lengthen your neck to look at the ceiling.

10. INHALE as you return to the erect posture with an Upward Salute.

11. EXHALE as you lower your hands to the floor behind your hips with your fingers forward. INHALE as you sit erect using your arm strength to extend your spine.

12. EXHALE bend forward pushing with your arms to expand your chest while

surrendering your head to the pull of gravity. Stay in this position for three breaths as you encourage your inner thighs to open.

13. INHALE come erect with your arms straightening to support your back. EXHALE remaining steady. This is the ideal time to remain steady and practice the Contemplation exercise.

14. INHALE extending your legs as you return to Stick pose. Remain still for sometime.

Notes for polishing your practice -

This posture begins to create a pyramid-like effect in the body – the energy of the body is well grounded in the pelvis and feet, thus creating a potentially stable base. This stable base tends to automatically enable energy to flow easily up through your body into the region of your heart and third eye, making it an excellent posture for pranayama and meditation.

Benefits -

The Hatha Yoga Pradipika chapter 1, sutra 55 states, "The Yogi who has thus overcome fatigue by practicing the asanas, should begin practice of purification of the subtle nerves, the nadis, manipulation of prana, pranayama, and mudras that introvert the subtle energies in order to generate a deeper meditation practice." [79]

The sequence of movements of the Bhadrasana Vinyasa can also be done from any sitting posture. This Vinyasa creates a thorough stretch for the groin muscles, the adductors, while simultaneously seeking to strengthen their antagonists the abductors, located at the deep outer sides of the hip. It can develop the tone and flexibility necessary to prepare your hips and back for sitting in meditation more comfortably.

One challenge for students is to develop their kinesthetic awareness of antagonist muscles working in harmony. Antagonist muscles are those that most directly oppose each other. For instance the hamstrings are antagonistic to the quadriceps with regard to knee flexion and knee extension, respectively. When one muscle stretches, that stretch will become more effective when the antagonist muscle is being consciously strengthened. Vice versa is also true. The student can begin this awareness by focusing upon the question – where do I feel the effects of the posture? Then answering the questions – What is the feeling? Is it a tight muscle attempting to stretch or a weakened muscle attempting to contract? By engaging this self-analysis process, you can create more leverage to free yourself from the bounds of limited mobility.

Auspicious Vinyasa
Bhadrasana
Mukunda Stiles © 2006

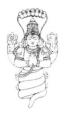

 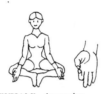 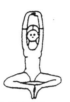

1- STICK
Dandasana
3 breaths

2- EXHALE - draw soles together; extend arms with hands in Jnana Mudra (Wisdom Seal) be still in Bhadrasana - Auspicious Pose

3- INHALE, arms up with outward fingerlock 3 breaths

4- EXHALE, hands to floor

5- INHALE, up repeat 4-5 three times.

   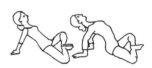

6- EXHALE, hold ankles then INHALE

7- EXHALE, forward bend elbows press knees open. Repeat 6-7, 3X.

8- INHALE, upward salute.

9- EXHALE, hand to floor behind hips. INHALE lift chest EXHALE extend head back

10- INHALE, arms up, sit erect

11- EXHALE, hands placed under hips. INHALE, then

12- EXHALE, bend forward. Stay with 3 full breaths.

13- INHALE, sit erect. EXHALE

14- INHALE to Stick pose take 3 breaths.

X - Vinyasas for Pitta

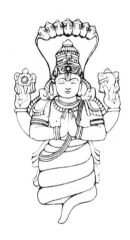

Sun Salutation — Surya Namaskar

The Sun Salutation or Surya Namaskar means "beautiful light I see myself as you." Surya means "beautiful light" and is one of the twelve mantra names for the sun. Namaskar is the singular form ("I am you") of the word Namaste meaning "I honor you." In the Vedic traditional practice of the Sun Salute, the sun was honored during at both sunrise and sunset. This practice deepens our humility; in it, we give gratitude for the force that sustains Life. Tantrik Yogis utilized this practice together with energetic breathing to take the sun's energy into their bodies. The advanced form of the practice involved directly experiencing the unity of the sun that is both outside and within your own body.

The practice of mantra as an invocation to an event is timeless. Mantra practice extends from the range of mental discipline to devotional practice. Among the most famous invocations to begin Sun Salutation practice is the following hymn from the Upanishads.

Asatoma sat-gamaya
Tamaso ma jyotir gamaya
Mrityor ma amritam gamaya
OM Ö *Shanti* Ö *Shanti* Ö   *Shantihi*

"O Lord, the essence of Light
Lead me from the unreal to the Real
From darkness to light
From death to Immortality
OM Ö *Peace* Ö *Peace* Ö *Peace"*
<u>Brihadaranyaka Upanishad</u> *I, iii, 28*

The Story of the Raja of Aund

The age of the practice is unknown. Some believe it to be of great antiquity, prior to the development of written language. The earliest writings, the Rig Veda, contain references to sun worship and are dated to the 3rd millennium BC. The Raja of Aundh (a former Indian state), Shrimant Pandit Pratinidhi, made Sun Salute a compulsory part of the physical training programs in schools throughout his kingdom during the 1940s. His subjects benefited greatly by improved health and vitality. He is quoted as saying "modern life is exceedingly wearing: the noise, the excitement, the hurry, the competition, irregular hours, hard study, anxieties, worry, lack of proper food and exercise, make a heavy tax on the constitution soon resulting in a breakdown of health. One can, however, be unaffected by these evils of modern civilization if one should perform the Surya-Namaskar exercise daily and take care of the diet and make proper use of sunshine and open air." [80]

Sun Salutation is the most widely known series of Yoga poses. All Yoga teachers present it in some variation. It is so highly regarded that there are entire books on this one practice. [81] According to the Ayurvedic physician Robert Svoboda, the "crest jewel of exercises is the Sun Salutation. . . The Sun Salutation is the supreme exercise because it balances and activates the body, controls and conditions the mind, and possesses a spiritual aspect as well. It is a salute to the sun, the source of our life. Even if you cannot work the Sun Salutation into your daily routine, no Vata is so disorganized, no Pitta is so busy, and no Kapha is so indolent that they cannot do some kind of exercise. If all else fails you can laugh. Laughter burns calories, improves lung function, oxygenates the blood, invites Prana into the system, releases endorphins, and strengthens the immune system. And it is so easy to do!" [82]

Contemplations (Dharana) -

Sun Salutation Mantras

The practice can also be done with a mantra for each of the twelve positions. The mantras are names and attributes of God. The ideal is to pause long enough in each asana to contemplate these qualities in the relationships you have with your inner teacher or Higher Power.

Aum Mitraya Namah	Mitra - friend
Aum Ravaye Namah	Ravi - "the shining twelve," containing all attributes
Aum Suryaya Namah	Surya – beautiful Light
Aum Bhanave Namah	Bhanu – brilliance and beauty of perception
Aum Khagaya Namah	Khaga – who moves in the sky
Aum Pusne Namah	Pushan – giver of strength
Aum Hiranyagarbhaya Namah	Hiranyagarbha – golden centered primordial egg
Aum Maricaye Namah	Marichi – Lord of the dawn
Aum Adityaya Namah	Aditya – Aditi is Mother of the twelve sun gods
Aum Savitre Namah	Savitri - beneficent feminine aspect of the sun
Aum Arkaya Namah	Arka - energy of the sun's rays
Aum Bhaskaraya Namah	Bhaskar – the Source that leads to illumination

After each round is complete the following mantra is then recited -
Aum Srisavitr-Suryanarayanaya Namah
I bow to the beneficent One, the Beautiful Light

Precautions –
While the Sun Salute is among the safest of sequences to practice, for those with back complaints there are three motions to modify in the instructions to follow.

First, is to exercise caution during standing forward bending poses by bending your knees. Second, Cobra pose is safest when done without use of arm strength as pushing the chest higher will stress the low back. Finally, although many schools of Yoga teach this sequence encouraging a deep standing backbend in postures 2 and 11, there is a potential for compression of the lumbar spinal discs, which can lead to pain. Therefore students are encouraged to lift their middle thoracic spine upwards, rather than extend it backwards. Increased flexibility alone and certainly that attained by straining your body is <u>not</u> Yoga.

Instructions -

1. Start in Samasthiti, Standing Steady, with your feet six inches apart, your palms together before your chest in prayer pose, Namaste. Close your eyes, take a series of deep breaths so that the flow of the breath is centered in the region of your heart, the inner sun. Imagine your inner sun rising as you breathe, spreading warmth throughout your body. Inwardly repeat this greeting given by T. Krishnamacharya, to your heart.

> *"I honor the divinity of my heart with all the*
> *warmth and cordiality of my mind."*

2. INHALE, arms extending forward and upward with palms forward thumbs overlapping in an upward pointing triangle (Shiva mudra), encouraging a mild backbend.

3. EXHALE, stretching forward in a sweeping forward bend to the Intensive Stretch pose (Uttanasana). At the end of the forward bend, your arms are relaxed and your forehead is close to your knees.

4. INHALE, bending your knees, your palms are placed outside your feet with finger tips in line with your toes. Stretch your right leg fully back allowing your knee to drop to the floor in a runner's stretch (also called the Equestrian pose – Ashwa Sanchalanasana). Your pelvis is down and forward to stretch your quadriceps. Expand your chest and look forward.

5. EXHALE, moving your left leg back as you lift your hips high while pushing your chest toward your knees. Lastly straighten your knees. This is Downward Facing Dog pose, Adho Mukha Svanasana. INHALE fully then on the next

6. EXHALE bend your knees coming briefly into cat pose with head up, then let your chest lead you to the floor, in cat bow. Hold your hips 6 inches from the floor as you form the Eight Part pose (Ashtangasana), touching sequentially knees, chest and then chin to the ground. Keep your elbows narrow.

7. INHALE squeeze your shoulder blades as you pull your chest forward onto the top of your feet, coming into the Cobra posture (Bhujangasana). Let the movement come from your spine to expand your chest fully.

8. EXHALE lift your hips high up and back coming to Downward Facing Dog

pose, straightening your legs at the end of the motion.

9.   INHALE returning your right foot between your hands with your toes placed even to your fingertips in the runner's stretch.

10.   EXHALE to the full forward bend, your left leg is brought forward so that your feet are aligned yet apart.

11.   INHALE, stretch your arms forward to initiate lifting up. The pull up of your arms will strengthen your middle back as you come up. Look up as you complete the upward and backward motion, tensing your buttocks.

12.   EXHALE. Palms come to heart position, Namaste.

REPEAT. On the next cycle, at position four, your left leg is brought back first, and again in position 9, your left leg is brought forward. This will balance the effects of stretching your quadriceps with strengthening your hip flexors. Two times through, with the reversed leg position, creates one cycle of Surya Namaskar.

Notes to polish your practice -

Among the common problems in Sun Salute is that when you establish the length of your extension into runner pose, that distance from hands to feet should be maintained throughout the sequence. Do not change your hand or foot position to make other postures easier. By maintaining this distance you will tend to receive the optimal extension of your spinal column which in turn will eliminate tension from your peripheral musculature.

Making the transition to return to the runner pose #9 from the Downward Facing Dog pose is often difficult for beginners. One helpful trick is to leave Down Facing Dog pose on your tiptoes so that your hips are raised as high as possible. This will allow the maximum length of swing so that the pendulum-like action of your leg can be brought forward more smoothly. In one quick motion bring your knee as close to your chest as possible. Simultaneously push your pelvis forward, maintaining close contact of your knee to your chest, so that in the final position your shin is perpendicular to the floor when your hips are fully pressed downward and forward.   If this does not permit your foot to come fully forward, then grasp your ankle and pull it up with a hopping motion to bring your toes aligned to your fingers.

Benefits -

The Sun Salute is the most beneficial Yoga sequence. It may be done slowly and gently to warm up the body or for a meditative inner focus. By deeply focusing upon deepening and lengthening the sound of Ujjaye breathing during the motions, the breath mantra can be heard and will increase introspection. Take at least 60 to 120 seconds for each half cycle.

The Sun Salute is a very powerful sequence of postures that both strengthens and extends the long muscles of the front and back of the body. It is a unique sequence that can stand alone without the need for other practices to maintain health. With consistent practice, it can increase limited hip and spinal flexibility. "The best flexibility gains can be made when the muscles are warm, immediately after a workout. The Sun Salute, because of its counterposing flexion and extension postures, is one of the most effective means of gaining flexibility." [83]

The ideal progression is to gradually increase your stamina by increasing both the number and the pace of your Sun Salutation cycles. In this manner the breath is extended so that instead of one motion per breath there will be up to three or four motions per breath. Initially, it is practiced a minimum of three or four times in sequence. For the first few days, concentrate on getting fullness in your movements. Later develop your breathing rhythm and flow. The breathing should be slow and deep in time with the flow of the poses. This may take a week or more of regular practice. Following that time, it can be increased to a total of six to ten repetitions, until your stamina is developed enough to maintain this flow, without becoming winded.

"With continued practice of the Sun Salute, the rib cage will reestablish its normal range of motion and flexibility, making deep diaphragmatic nasal breathing - the preferred breathing technique both during exercise and at rest - easier to perform." [84]

Gradually, in the second month, it can be increased to twenty or twenty-five repetitions, at which point the effect on the heart and cardiovascular system are at a pace to be able to maintain their health and vigor. Done regularly, twenty repetitions will tone your body and help to reduce excess weight. When done with full continuous breathing, each sequence should take approximately one minute for a half cycle. It can be done more vigorously over a 10 - 20 minute period for an aerobic effect to strengthen the cardiovascular system. According to the yoga staff of Dr. Dean Ornish's Program for Reversing Heart Disease, this is the most beneficial exercise for their heart patients. The patients who do the best in their recovery from heart disease are those who have extended their Yoga practices extend beyond 75 minutes. The emphasis within the poses can also be modified for developing muscular stamina by having a brief pause in each asana.

Once you have developed the discipline of regular practice for six continuous months, you are encouraged to modify the practice. The awakening to the spirit of guidance from your Prana is most likely to arise from this. Often dance-like spontaneous motions of body or breath (Kriyas) will arise from this experience. The inner Shakti of an awakened Prana will guide you to beautiful, unpredictable yet safe variations.

Variation

My spiritual teacher, Swami Muktananda Paramahansa, taught an intensive variation on the Sun Salute, which he recommended for teenagers and yoga teachers to practice at gradually increased speed. This can be safely achieved after one achieves the stamina to do twenty rounds slowly and rhythmically coordinated with their breath, (which should take 20 minutes). Teachers should increase to one hundred times or fifty rounds of sun salute, doing it as fast as possible, so that the rhythm is not at breath rate (one inhale or exhale per movement), but rather doing the entire cycle on 2 or 3 breaths. In this manner, the breath is steady and just as long as normal.

With regular practice, this can be done in about fifteen to twenty minutes. It has a tremendously strong aerobic effect on the cardiovascular system, producing similar effects as running or swimming, without their downside.

Three Methods of Practice According to Ayurvedic Guidelines

As is mentioned in the chapter on Ayurvedic asanas, there are three main methods of approach to Yoga practices. To promote flexibility, sensitivity and to balance the air/ether quality of Vata, Vinyasa practices are ideal when performed slowly, deliberately, rhythmically with ujjaye pranayama. In this method of practicing the Sun Salutation, practice will take 60 seconds to perform one cycle or half a round. Emphasis is upon moving slowly and deliberately concentrating on the internal wave motion and glottal sound of the ujjaye breathing pattern. This is the way to practice during the winter. This manner promotes peace as it heightens sensitivity to hidden thoughts and feelings as it arouses insight. It also releases fear and curbs anxiety when practiced regularly. An understanding of your attainable aspirations comes into focus and your burdens are lifted.

The second method involves a focus on promoting vitality, energy, and heat sufficient to balance the fire/water quality of Pitta. There is little attention paid to the breath except to allow it to move freely. The pacing will tend to be faster than in the previous method. Emphasis is upon moving with vigor and enthusiasm to generate body heat and/or sensitivity to energy flow within the body. This practice is most suitable for early morning hours of the summer and winter. It redirects frustration, anger, and excess sexuality transforming them into creativity and abundant enthusiasm. Swami Muktananda's method falls into this category.

The third method promotes strength, purifies the physical body, and develops stamina that balances the earth/water quality of Kapha. Attention is focused upon the sense of strength developed during each posture and cumulatively over repetitive sequences. The amount of time taken to practice a sequence is longest for this method. This is the ideal attitude for spring and fall practice. Elongation of the body is promoted by the strength to lift upward against the force of gravity. A strong physique is created from a focus on toning, not from stretching. The exhale is encouraged to be longer than inhale and periodically released through the mouth with a sigh sound. This method helps to release sadness and lethargy and to bring normalize weight for your physique. It promotes courage, hopefulness, faithfulness, and humility.

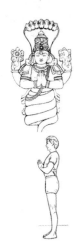

Sun Salutation
Surya Namaskar

*I honor the Divinity of my Heart
with all the warmth and cordiality of my mind.*
Namaste (from Sri Krishnamacharya)

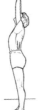

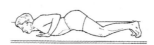
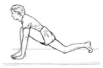

1 - EXHALE
Tadasana -
Mountain Pose

2 - INHALE
Urdhva Namaskar
Upward Salute

3 - EXHALE
Uttanasana -
Intensive Stretch

4 - INHALE
Ashwa sanchalanasana
Equestrian or runner pose
right leg back 1st time

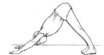
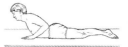

5 - EXHALE
   Adho Mukha Svanasana -
   Down Facing Dog Pose

6 - EXHALE
   Ashtangasana -
   Eight Part Pose – Cat Bow

7 - INHALE
   Bhujangasana -
   Cobra Pose

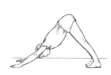
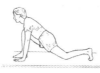

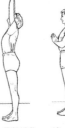

8 – EXHALE

9 - INHALE
right leg forward 1ˢᵗ time

10 - EXHALE   11 - INHALE   12 - EXHALE
Namaskar

Cobra — Bhujangasana Vinyasa

Bhujangasana

The Cobra pose resembles the movements of a serpent in a ready, attentive pose about to strike its prey or protect its territory. Our shoulder blades are brought back; flaring open our chest muscles from the uplifting action of the diaphragm. The open diaphragm gives the appearance of a cobra's hood flared open in an attitude of alertness. The sternum is lifted high and brought forward in an assertive manner. This strengthens the major back and neck muscles. The head is held level with the eyes looking straight ahead.

Contemplation (Dharana) -

The story of the serpent, the snake, is the story of man's struggle for uncovering his eternal True Self. The serpent knows what we seek to know. In India it is known as the Goddess Kundalini, in the Hebrew Torah as the serpent, and in ancient Egypt the snake lived beyond the eternity of change. According to the third chapter of the book of Genesis, the serpent was cursed to crawl below all other creatures on the earth, but it possessed the ability to discriminate between good and evil. According to the Egyptian Book of the Dead, the snake understands life and the nature of change.

Inevitability of Change from the Egyptian Book of the Dead

The Story of Becoming the Snake

"The story goes that change is inevitable. So it must be that having eaten dust and rotting flesh, the snake comes to know in his own skin the secrets of change. Through the deceit of death I grow wise in the illusions of time. To change, I grow beyond myself, leaving the papery sheath that once was what I was. I live alone and make my changes in secret. I know the smell of fear, of death, of innocence. . . I lick the wisdom of air and dust. I know the earth, sky and men. I wrap myself around the legs of life. By the enmity of others I learn empathy with all creatures. I lie down in darkness and learn the art of subtlety. I rear and strike in surprise. . . I lie down and change and rise and grow old and lie down and change and rise. I demand neither fear nor pity. I know what you cannot see. It is not pride that keeps me solitary. In your hands the honey of my mouth turns to poison. It is mere survival - yours and mine.

Change is eternity." [85]

Precautions –

All backbending poses need to be approached with caution. For anyone with any low back conditions – sciatica, lumbar disc herniation, or sacroiliac sprain – the backbending postures should be modified so that they produce the most comfort and spinal elongation. Anyone with a weak back, strain in their sacroiliac, or their lumbar region should not hold these poses longer than 30 seconds or 3 breaths. Rather they should do repetitions of the pose to develop lumbar stamina. One breath up and one breath down per movement, with a resting breath between each movement is sufficient. The student is cautioned to maintain a pelvic tilt, pressing the pubic area into the floor during each backbending exertion so that compression of the lumbar spine is minimized.

It is common for women to be intuitive and know that Cobra pose should be eliminated at some point after the first trimester of pregnancy. Without attempting the poses they will realize that it would put too much pressure on their abdomen and lower back. It's better for them to do either the Sunbird pose with the Sun Salute or to work with the Sunbird Vinyasa which provides similar strengthening benefits to the lumbar spine and hip region without the risk of the Cobra.

All back bends are stimulating to the sympathetic nervous system, causing a mild increase in blood pressure and heart rate. The regulator for this increase is the baroreceptors located in the wall of the common carotid arteries of the neck and the wall of the descending aorta. In both cases the pressure regulator or baroreceptorbarroreceptor sensor is located where the arteries branch. By stretching these locations, as in backbends, blood pressure is increased. The increases will be minimal, and are of no cause for concern, unless the postures are held longer than is given in these instructions.

During all backbends breathing can become labored. It is especially important to encourage evenness and fullness of breath during these postures so that sensitivity and relaxation of effort can be optimized during your exertions. Students who are overzealous in backbends will benefit from prolonged stays in Downward Facing Dog pose as this can balance the strength of the upper and lower back muscles.

The main effect to seek in all asanas is an elongation of your spine while maintaining natural spinal curves. Encourage yourself to elongate forward from your lumbar spine simultaneously reaching backward from your hips and legs. Done in this manner these movements will result in a spinal decompression and heightened sense of vitality.

Instructions –

1. Begin lying face down, legs together, and hands beside your chest with your fingers forward. Keep your elbows drawn in and down. Take a series of full wave breaths, and then contract your inner thigh muscles to pull your legs more firmly together.

2. INHALE and using only your back muscles pull your torso forward from the floor as you raise your upper body, coming into Cobra posture.

3. EXHALE slowly and return to the floor. REPEAT steps 2 to 3 three times, each time continuing to elongate your ribcage away from your waist.

4. INHALE and bring your hands behind your back, interlacing your fingers, and draw your shoulder blades together. EXHALE fully then as you

5. INHALE raise up your upper body with your shoulders and arms pulled back along your legs. EXHALE down. Repeat steps 4 to 5 three times.

6. INHALE as you place your palms on the floor beside your chest. INHALE as you separate your feet six inches bringing your toes forward so your knees are lifted.

7. EXHALE and push your hips up and back, while pressing your chest towards your knees. Lower your chin towards your chest. Do not straighten your legs until your back and arms feel fully extended to elevate your hips. Then slowly straighten your knees to complete the Downward Facing Dog pose, Adho Mukha Svanasana. Stay with a lengthening effort for six full breaths.

8. EXHALE and lower your body straight to the floor, separating your legs hips width, placing your hands palm up under or beside your thighs, whichever is more comfortable.

9. INHALES as you stretch your right leg back and lift it up in the Half Locust pose, Ardha Salabhasana. Raise your head and shoulders to a comfortable level. EXHALE down.

10. PAUSE as you open your legs hip's width. Repeat the pose three times, alternating sides as you lift.

11. INHALE stretch both legs out and lift them hip width apart to come into full Locust pose. Stay for three full breath cycles.

12. EXHALE lowering your legs then turn your toes under, hands beside your chest. INHALE then

13. EXHALE pushing your hips up and back slowly extending your legs into Downward Facing Dog pose. Stay for 6 breaths.

14. EXHALE press your hips backward as you lower your knees to the floor, resting your hips on your heels. Relax your body over your thighs in the Fetal pose, Garbhasana. Relax further by allowing your arms and head to drop forward into the floor. Stay for six deep breaths.

15. INHALE as you stretch your legs back, laying face down and opening your thighs with your feet turned inward. Stretch one arm forward, bending at your elbow to create a cradle to rest your eyes in the fold of that elbow. Bring your other arm over the top so that your elbows are above each other. Adjust your arms until there is no light entering your eyes and then soften so you can relax deeply in the Crocodile pose, Makarasana, staying for a minimum of one minute.

Benefits -

The Cobra Vinyasa is composed of two primary backbending postures – the Cobra pose and the Locust pose. In both positions, the lower back and the buttocks are strengthened. Cobra can be done using your arms or not. When it is done using arm strength, it strengthens the latissimus and trapezius, the more superficial muscles of the back. When done without the aid of arm strength it strengthens the deep layers of muscles along your spinal column, the erector spinae. This is usually a more demanding variation. While the Locust posture also strengthens these muscles in reverse, i.e. from bottom to top, its primary effect is strength to the hip extensor muscles – the gluteus maximus and hamstrings.

The backbending poses are interspersed with Downward Facing Dog pose which serves as a forward bending counterpose to decompress the spinal column and lengthen the hamstrings. By allowing your head to hang in this posture your neck also lengthens as it releases cervical compression. The series is a mild yet stimulating sequence that restores Pitta to bring about healthy vitality and digestion.

Spiritual Awakening

In all mystical traditions, it is believed that there is an innate Spirit seeking to guide each of us to realize their potential. Sometimes the search for Spirit is done in the dream state, sometimes through the awesomeness of Nature, or in this case through yoga. Whatever is done for Spiritual evolution never goes to waste it will always produce beneficial results even in the unforeseen future.

The Cobra pose is described in the Gheranda Samhita II, 37 which says, "The practice of Bhujangasana removes all ailments, invigorates the body and awakens the Serpent-Goddess (Kundalini)." However, it is highly unlikely that you might experience an awakening of your spiritual energy, the Shakti Kundalini, through Yoga postures. Nonetheless, it is important to know something of the signs of true awakening. Yoga postures may provoke short-lived mystical experiences such as energy in the spine, visions, or heat coursing through your body uncontrollably. These are not signs of a Kundalini awakening and will typically end within minutes of completing the stimulating practice. There is no danger in these short-lived experiences, except one's fear of the unknown. If fear is raised, then consulting a teacher who has experienced a true spiritual awakening may be of great comfort.

In contrast, a true spiritual awakening is a long-term process in which the experiences continue to take on a constellation of expressions over a long period of time. These are normally preceded by an intense desire for change, a spiritual quest, or extremes of emotional or physical suffering. Often during these preliminary periods, the student is praying to God or the Unknown for relief from some form of suffering.

Cobra Vinyasa
Bhujangasana
Mukunda Stiles © 2007

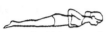 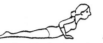 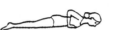 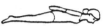

1- Begin with legs pressed together elbows in & up

2- INHALE, raise the trunk without aid from the arms Cobra Pose – Bhujangasana

3- EXHALE, slowly return to the floor. Repeat 2-3, 3 times.

4- INHALE, interlace fingers with shoulders together. EXHALE, then

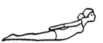 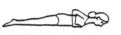 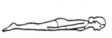

5- INHALE, raise torso. EXHALE, lower Repeat 4-5, 3 times

6- EXHALE, lower torso INHALE placing hands under shoulders. Toes forward, then

7- EXHALE, push hips up and back into Down Face Dog Pose - Adho Mukha Svanasana. Stay for 6 breaths

8- EXHALE, lower to floor placing hands under thighs.

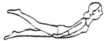 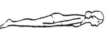 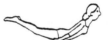 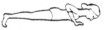

9- INHALE, raise right leg with straight knee. EXHALE down & repeat alternating legs, three times.

10- PAUSE, down to floor feet open one foot.

11- INHALE, raise open legs, stay for 3 breaths Locust pose - Salabhasana

12- EXHALE, lower to floor & place hands under shoulders. INHALE then

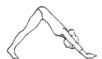 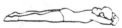

13- EXHALE, push hips up to Dog pose.

14- EXHALE, lower knees then torso to Fetal pose - Garbhasana

15- Rest, lay forward, placing the head in the bend of one elbow, legs open, toes in. Crocodile pose - Makarasana

Sunbird — Chakravakasana Vinyasa

Chakravakasana

Chakravakasana gets its name from a mythological goose of reddish color that appears at sunrise. According to ancient myth the Sunbird flies to earth each morning, bringing with it the warmth and color of the morning sun. Brahma and Sarasvati ride on this goose as the vehicle that transports them and their power of creativity to their devotees.

In recent times, a reddish colored goose called the "bar-headed goose (anser indicus) has been seen flying at 30,000 feet, just below the troposphere, on their annual migration from Tibet and over the Himalayas to India. To survive at such altitudes, where the temperature is minus 80° C and it is difficult to absorb enough oxygen, the birds have evolved to cope with thee conditions. It is estimated that in flight their hearts beat at 400 times per minute." [86] This flight pattern is higher than any other bird has been spotted. Their physiology has somehow developed an ability to adapt to a lowered level of Pitta and extremes of Kapha. This practice helps restore adaptability to the extremes of heat and cold.

Dharana (Contemplation)

Adi Shankara and the Sunbird story

Early one fall morning, young Adi Shankar was up as was his usual custom, before sunrise. He set out to tend his father's rice field when he happened upon a beautiful large red goose near his home. The startled great bird let out a sudden cry as he leapt into the air, which made young Shankar stand dead in his tracks. He remained motionless for some time yet his eyes were fixed upon the flight of the ruddy goose, which seemed to fly straight into the majestic orange harvest sun. As it moved farther away it appeared to grow smaller against the background of the perfectly circular rising sun. The bird merged into the sun becoming like a concentrated pregnant spot, a bindu. Shankara's awareness went with the Chakravak bird and merged into the universal field of consciousness. This experience deepened until his mind could no longer contain itself. In liberating his mind he entered that state of pure consciousness without thought, the fundamental field from which all perception arises.

As a result of his experience, Shankar later became a Sannyas (renunciate monk), creating the first order of Indian Swamis. A Swami is one who takes a vow of permanent renunciation of the sense of "I" as one's ego identity. He formulated the teachings that are known today as Advaita Vedanta, the science of non-dualism. Its principal teaching is that "There is only One." Many of Adi Shankaracharya's writings are left to us as insightful commentaries on the search for meaning in life.

Shankara's experience is also that of the great Sufi poet Rumi, who wrote about seeing and being that great bird.

> What I want is to see your face
> in a tree, in the sun coming out,
> in the air. . . .
> I'm tied of cowards.
> I want to live with lions.
> With Moses. . . .
> Last night,
> A great teacher went from door to door
> With a lamp. ""He who is not to be found
> Is the one I'm looking for."
> But Love plays
> and is the music played.
> Let that musician
> Finish this poem. Shams,
> I am a water bird
> flying into the sun. [87]

Precautions –
The Hero Pose, Virasana, requires full flexibility of the knees and ankles simultaneously. Many people lack this combination so follow this advice. If your ankles or knees do not permit you to sit comfortably on your shins in Hero pose, adjust your posture by placing a pad behind your knees to open the space of your knee joint. This will lessen the demand on your quadriceps to stretch. A pad can also be placed between the top of the arch and the floor in the event of stiff ankles. If these adjustments are insufficient to make the pose comfortable, then do the series by beginning and ending in position two, an upright kneeling pose. It is most important that you allow yourself to be comfortable in a modified position, rather than straining your body to force it into the "proper position."

Instructions –
1. Begin by sitting in Hero pose, Virasana, with your feet and thighs close together or touching. Rest your right palm in your left with the tips of your thumbs lightly touching forming the Seal of Meditation (Dhyana Mudra), a hand gesture that promotes expanded consciousness.   Close your eyes and take a series of slow wave breaths.
2. INHALE and sweep your arms sideways until they come together overhead in the upward salutation (Urdhva Namaste) while bringing your hips up so that your torso comes into a straight line with your thighs.

3.   EXHALE as you lower your hips back down to your heels, then gently bend forward from your hips so your body will rest on your thighs with your arms relaxed forward in the Fetal Pose, Darnikasana, with your arms relaxed in front.

4.   INHALE and slide your body forward coming to rest on your forearms in a modified Cat Pose. Adjust your arms and legs until they are parallel. EXHALE round your back upward while allowing your head to come toward your chest.

5.   INHALE as you stretch your right leg back on the floor then lift it above hip height and look up. Keep your knee firm and hips level. This is the Sunbird Pose, Chakravakasana.

6.   EXHALE and return to the previous position, gazing between your hands.

7.   INHALE stretch your left leg out then lift it as you look up. EXHALE return to the previous pose.

8.   INHALE stretch your hips back toward heels, while your arms extend forward with your hea lifted. Encourage a stretch from your hips to your fingertips.

9.   EXHALE relax lowering your forehead and elbows to the floor returning to the Fetal Pose.

10. INHALE pelvic tilt your lower pelvis forward to roll your spine up, sitting on your heels in Hero Pose with your arms raised into Upward Salute, Urdhva Namaste.

11. EXHALE lowering your arms, returning your hands to the Seal of Meditation.
     REPEAT the cycle at least three times continuously or until a smooth flow can be created.

Benefits -

Physically this sequence brings the knees and hip joints to full flexion and extension. These motions both strengthen and stretch your quadriceps and hamstrings. The motions into and out of the Sunbird Pose extend the hips which will strengthen the buttock muscles and the lumbar region. These motions are beneficial for persons with weak or stiffness in their lower backs as they provide a safe approach to strengthening and flexing the lower back. Most backbending exercises involve the use of the arms strength. The downside of these poses is that they can overpower the delicate deep muscles of the spinal column and cause strain.

The major emphasis in the sequence needs to remain upon extending the spinal column. I cannot emphasize this enough. While all yogasanas are to be done with spinal extensions, this particular sequence is more likely to produce the feeling of the decompression we are seeking for Yoga Therapy purposes. Learning how to undulate your spine up from the Fetal pose to Hero (positions 9 to 10) can greatly enhance the opening of the lumbar spine. By the development of a strong pelvic tilt to begin the motion, you will develop the rectus abdominis sequentially from the lower to upper segments. By taking time to isolate the feelings of tone to each individual segment of your abdomen, you can develop the sensitivity to truly lessen the stress you carry.

Pregnant women may find this posture relieves lower back strains, which is common during the second and third trimesters. They are especially encouraged to flex their spine both ways that are described in position four. In both cases it is important to bring the foot level to the height of the head and not above this height as the increased motion may aggravate your lower back rather than relieve it.

The Sunbird Vinyasa can be done as a meditative routine that gracefully moves your body through the contrasts of forward and backward bending. This effect is most easily obtained by doing dynamic steady repetitions of the series until the desired effect arises. It has a mildly heating effect thus promoting a gentle stimulation of Pitta, while tending toward balancing Vata.

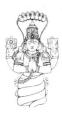

Sunbird Vinyasa
Chakravakasana
Mukunda Stiles © 2007

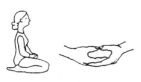
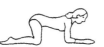
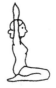
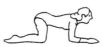
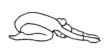
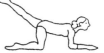

1- Hero Pose -Virasana
Sit on heels, thighs strongly
squeezing. Hands in Dhyana
"Meditation Mudra".

2- INHALE, raise onto
knees arms overhead.

3- EXHALE, sit back
onto heels..

Same EXHALE, bend
forward to Fetal Pose
- Garbhasana

4- INHALE, move forward
resting on forearms with
neutral head.   EXHALE,
cat tuck-- back up, head down.
(Not shown).

5- INHALE, raise right leg
knee straight. Sunbird pose
- Chakravakasana

6- EXHALE, back to
neutral spine.

7- INHALE, raise left leg
with knee straight
EXHALE, leg down.

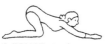

8- INHALE, stretch arms
forward, hips back, head up -
Extended Fetal Pose.

9- EXHALE, relax head
hips and elbows down in
Fetal Pose.

10- INHALE, raise arms
and sit on heels.

11- EXHALE, lower
palms up in
Meditation
Mudra; repeat 3X.

XI - Vinyasas for Kapha

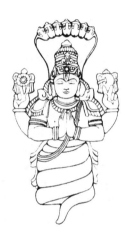

Warrior — Virabhadrasana Vinyasa

Virabhadrasana

Virabhadra is the name of a legendary warrior created by Shiva's wrath. This Vinyasa combines both open and closed hip standing poses that challenge the strength and flexibility of the lower back and hips. These poses can empower or overpower students depending upon the teacher's sensitivity to their student's abilities and limitations. Done in the sequence of this Vinyasa, the poses are more approachable and digestible then done in isolation.

Contemplation (Dharana)

Siva Virabhadra Story (transforming wrath) [88]

Daksha was a great and powerful Tantrik Yogi, whose power had given him a swollen head, believing himself to being a god. He married Prasuti, the daughter of Manu, the universal lawgiver, and had 16 beautiful daughters. The youngest, Sati, became the second wife of Shiva-Bhava, one of Shiva's eight forms, known for his serenity and complete detachment from the world. As the ruler of transformation, Shiva had a special love for death and rebirth, and could often be found doing his Tantrik practices at the cremation grounds.

One day Daksha decided to throw a big party in his own honor in order to impress the world with the supernatural powers he had gained through mastery of the sacrificial fire, yagna. But he did not want to invite his son-in-law Shiva because of his "unclean practices." Daksha became indignant at the thought of Shiva's dirty body covered with ashes from the cremation ground disrupting his ceremony. He didn't want him anywhere near his special guests, so he did not include Shiva among the gods to whom he offered the yagna. Big mistake!!!

Sati was by nature pious and dutiful, and so her father's exclusion of her husband from the ceremony humiliated her and left her despondent for days. She could not conceive of a way that could reconcile the two major men in her life. Out of her depression, accompanied by morose and suicidal thoughts, she threw herself into the fire that was to consume the sacred offerings. News of this shocking event soon reached Shiva's first wife, Parvati. (Bad news travels fast, even in the days before satellite TV.) When she told Shiva, initially he was unmoved. Out of empathy for Parvati's distress, he felt compelled to take revenge. It seemed that Shiva had only two emotions, serenity and violent rage. In his shift into a destructive rage, Shiva tore the hair from his matted head and threw it on the ground.

Out of Shiva's wrath sprang a powerful warrior, Virabhadra, with three eyes, four arms, and tusks protruding from his mouth. He wore a garland of skulls and held a trident in one right hand and a club in one left hand. His other hands displayed the mudra signs of compassion: Abhaya Mudra (a gesture capable of dispelling fear) with an open palm facing up, and Varada Mudra (a gesture of bestowing boons) with an open palm facing down. Virabhadra was sent to destroy the fire ceremony. He appeared like a hurricane, destroyed the sacrifice, and massacred the unrighteous complacent bystanders. The virtuous guests fled to seek Shiva's grace and forgiveness for their foolishness. Once Daksha was found, he was beheaded by Virabhadra, who threw the severed head into the Yagna's fires.

Shiva's revenge was complete. Later that night Sati spoke to Shiva in a dream, imploring him to give her father back his life. Shiva consented to restore his life but not his head. This he replaced with the head of a ram. The karma complete, Sati could be reborn as Uma, the Goddess of the Himalayas. She lived many years in seclusion in the remote valleys and caves of the Himalayas until completing her spiritual training. Then she once again became Shiva's second bride. And they lived happily ever after.

Precautions –

Do not do this Vinyasa if you have an acute knee injury. However, collectively the poses making up the variations of Virabhadrasana are quite beneficial for recovering a healthy knee following injuries. Be especially careful to make sure your knees are properly positioned. If you don't feel stable in the standing poses increase the side-to-side width of your foot placement. This adjustment is especially beneficial in relieving strains to your inner knees and sacroiliac region.

Instructions

1. Stand in an erect Standing Steady posture (Samasthiti).
2. EXHALE and step wide apart so your feet are three feet apart.
3. INHALE stretch your arms out and overhead interlacing your fingers.
4. EXHALE form an outward finger lock as you turn your hips to face squarely to your left. Check your foot position: your left foot is pointing straight ahead and your right foot angles out slightly (2 o'clock). INHALE and extend you spine, lifting up out of your waist.
5. EXHALE bending your left knee until your shin is perpendicular to the floor. This is Warrior I. Hold the position for three steady breaths. Then on the next
6. EXHALE lower your arms to the side, parallel with the floor, palms facing down.
7. INHALE bring your palms to your heart in the Namaste gesture. EXHALE staying still.
8. INHALE your arms up overhead into an outward finger lock as you straighten your left knee.
9. EXHALE forward bend, lowering your hands towards your left ankle. INHALE extend your spine forward.

10. EXHALE lowering your head so that your forehead is closer to your shin. Repeat the last two motions three times, gradually lengthening your spine to comfortable capacity as you lower your hands toward the floor. This is the Side Stretch pose, Parsvottanasana. Stay here for 3 breaths.
11. INHALE lift your torso to an upright position with arms overhead. EXHALE lower arms parallel to the floor at shoulder height and at the same time rotate your torso to face front. Form an open hip position with the left foot at 9 o'clock and the right foot at 10 o'clock. INHALE fully lengthening your spine and arms.
12. EXHALE move your torso as a unit from your hip joint and bring your left hand to rest on your mid-shin. Steady yourself for three breaths in the Extended Triangle position, Utthita Trikonasana. If you can maintain cervical alignment INHALE rotate your head to look at your extended right thumb, palm facing front.
13. INHALE and lift up to standing, resuming position #11.
14. EXHALE bend your left knee until your shin comes perpendicular to the floor with your torso remaining vertical to form Warrior II, Virabhadrasana. Stay for three breaths.
    INHALE return to center standing position with fingers interlaced overhead (position #3). Then repeat all the poses on the right side.
15. After completing the postures on both sides return to Standing Steady pose, and remain there to feel the effects of the Warrior Vinyasa. Lie down in Savasana and feel the benefits.

Notes for polishing your practice -

The muscles of the hips are intricate and they interact with each other in various combinations that tend to both strengthen and bind the pelvic girdle to the spinal column. To help facilitate a balance of stamina yet freedom to these dynamic forces of the spinal column, I encourage doing micro-movements with the basic four asanas of this sequence. They consist of repetitively doing pelvic tilt and thrust, sideways pelvic swing (lifting up on one hip socket while descending the other), and drawing a circle with the pelvis. By repeating these motions 6-10 times in each position you will be creating freedom of the joints and stamina in the deeper muscular tissues. These micro motions may also bring up emotional patterns held by restricted pelvic mobility. This benefit can be pursued in individual Ayurvedic Yoga Therapy sessions if you are not comfortable giving expression to these emotions and energies in class.

Opening your feet to an increasingly wider stance is a great way to challenge the capacity of your body to adapt to change. Keep in mind that the increased stance will place increased pressure at both your hip joints and your sacral ligaments. So these are beneficial only if you have no concerns for these delicate regions of your anatomy. Increasing the width of your base or the depth of your pelvis is not recommended until you have spent time with the micro-movements to free up the pelvis.

Benefits –

Standing positions with both open and closed hip variations powerfully work the muscles of the thighs and buttocks. These postures provide balance to hips, pelvis, and spine through the strong opposing movements of the closed versus the opened hip positions. By giving plenty of time with these poses Yoga students can make wonderful strides in their capacity to do comfortable seated poses. This series can definitely increase your comfort in all forms of sitting, while the floor poses alone cannot make the difference in ease of sitting. The Warrior pose, especially variation one, dramatically opens the respiratory muscles and begins to enhance their stamina. Overtime increase your holding time of each of these primary postures to optimize this benefit.

The Warrior is a powerful image and certainly one of the most dynamic postures in Yoga. The Warrior is especially beneficial in creating strength and stamina by challenging your endurance. The sequence includes both open and closed hip variations of Virabhadrasana. The open hip positions (Warrior II and Extended Triangle) create a powerful stretching of the adductors, which comprise the greatest bulk of the thigh as well as toning the outer thigh and hip. Moving between these two poses is beneficial for lessening the muscular tensions associated with bowed legs and knock-knees as well as weak ankles, particularly fallen arches or flat feet. Also stretching the inner thighs (adductors) is beneficial for runners as an important factor in preventing injuries to these muscles as well as their posterior neighbors, the hamstrings.

The closed hip positions (Warrior I and Side Stretch) reverse the effects of open hip positions, thus strengthening the groin (adductors) while stretching the outer thighs and buttocks (hip extensors and external rotators).

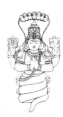

Warrior Vinyasa
Virabhadrasana
Mukunda Stiles © 2007

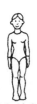 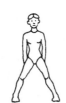 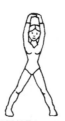 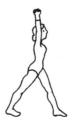 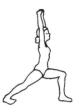

1- Steady Pose Samasthiti

2- EXHALE, legs open 3 feet

3- INHALE, arms sweep outward and fingers interlace

4- EXHALE, form an outward fingerlock as you twist body to the left. INHALE lengthening spine then

5- EXHALE, bend left knee to Warrior Pose Virabhadrasana I INHALE then

6- EXHALE, lower arms parallel to floor, palms down.

7- INHALE, Namaste to your heart. Then after an EXHALE

8- INHALE raise arms to outward fingerlock, straighten leg

9- EXHALE, bend forward, hands to shin. INHALE extend your spine

10- EXHALE, lower head to Side Stretch Pose - Parsvottanasana

11- INHALE up. EXHALE twist to front then INHALE lengthening spine

12- EXHALE, to side in Extended Triangle -Utthita Trikonasana

13- INHALE, come up

14- EXHALE, bend left thigh to Warrior Pose II INHALE up to #3 then repeat series on right

15- INHALE, come to Samasthiti

Bridge — Setubandhasana Vinyasa

Setubandhasana

The Bridge Vinyasa is a preparatory sequence for doing the Shoulderstand posture and Vinyasa safely. It builds the upper back strength and flexibility. It is composed of variations of the Bridge pose followed by a twist to counterpose the sequence of backbending.

Precautions –

Occasionally some students experience knee pain from doing repetitions of the Bridge pose. Normally the problem is due to losing the vertical alignment of your shins. Your knees are to be kept directly above your ankles. Also check to be certain that your feet are pointing straight ahead. One exception to this alignment is for students with tibial torsion. This is a genetic postural misalignment in which the knees do not align with the shins and the feet splay out the side while the knee is pointing straight ahead. For students with this condition, the knees are stressed by aligning the feet. They will be more comfortable in the Bridge poses with their feet turned outward yet they should still maintain the knee above ankle alignment.

For most beginners, doing many or prolonged Bridge poses can flatten the cervical curve. Unless the shoulders have both strength and stamina to maintain scapular adduction with shoulder external rotation in the position, the neck will be in a weight-bearing position. Without shoulder rotation, there can be numbness from the occlusion of the brachial plexus. This region is composed of blood vessels and nerves that exit the cervical spine, shoulders and extend down the arms. The result of this would be loss of feeling or tingling in the arms or hands. If the shoulder joints can open fully, then the armpits will remain open, giving space for these vessels to pass unrestricted. Ideally the shoulders and outer arm muscles (trapezius, posterior deltoids, and triceps) will provide the support for the weight of the entire upper body, which is a necessary prelude to supporting the entire body weight during the full Shoulderstand pose. When this combination of openness and postural strength is achieved the cervical curve will remain naturally arched off the floor.

Instructions -

1 - Begin by lying on your back with your knees bent, feet open comfortably close to your hips and hip width apart. Rest your arms at your sides, palms up, with your shoulders turned outward. Keep your neck and head still throughout the sequence.

2 - With an INHALE, lift your pelvis so that your torso makes a straight line from shoulders to your knees. Keep your knees over your ankles. Remain steady for three breaths.

3 - EXHALE lowering your hips to the floor. PAUSE after the exhale and reach your arms overhead shoulder width apart with your palms up.

4 - INHALE as you lift your hips stretching your arms along the floor. Stay for three breaths.

5 - EXHALE lowering your hips. PAUSE after the exhale and bring your hands palm down onto your inner thighs, encourage your shoulders to round forward and down.

6 - INHALE as you lift your hips reaching your arms down your legs. Stay for three breaths.

7 - EXHALE as you lower your hips. PAUSE and form an outward finger lock with your palms above your chest.

8 - INHALE as you lift your hips stretch your arms up toward the ceiling. Take three breaths.

9 - EXHALE lower your hips. PAUSE opening your arms to the floor shoulder height with your palms upward.

10 - INHALE raising your hips as you reach sideways. Take three breaths.

11 - EXHALE to lower your body. PAUSE lowering your hands beside your hips with your left leg straight.

12 - INHALE raise your hips keeping them level as you reach out through your left leg. Steady yourself for three breaths. EXHALE lowering your hips and reverse legs, repeat.

13 - Keep your right leg straight, placing the left foot on the right knee. INHALE fully, and then EXHALE slide your hips 6" to the left as you rotate your hips so that your outer right hip rests on the floor. Your bent left knee will come close to the floor in the Abdominal Twist pose - Jathara Parivartanasana. Turn your head to gaze at the left hand and take 6 full breaths. INHALE as you come back onto your back, then reverse legs.

14 - EXHALE bending both knees toward your chest coming into Energy Freeing pose - Apanasana. Grip your upper shins with both hands and pull until you feel your lower back stretching. Stay in this counter stretch for a minimum of 6 full breaths.

15 - INHALE and extend your arms and legs to Relaxation pose, Savasana, and rotate your consciousness through all the naturally arising "currents of sensation" for 1-2 minutes.

Notes to polish your practice –

During all the Bridge pose variations, concentrate on using your hip strength equal to the effort of your thighs. Once you have memorized the sequence, you can make it more challenging by rolling the spine as you move in and out of each variation. Doing this Rolling Bridge pose variation creates a powerful tone to your abdominal muscles and to the layers of your deep back musculature, the erector spinae.

While doing the Abdominal Twist, seek to maintain a mild backbend by making an arch in your lower back. With an exhale, arch your back and place your right hand on your outer left knee, twisting it toward the floor, keeping your shoulders level to the floor.   Fully rotate your head until your ear is close to the floor.

Benefits –

This Vinyasa is composed of several arm motions in conjunction with hip extension. Each of the arm positions changes the pressure applied to the neck and shoulder region as the hips are raised and lowered. This helps to warm up the neck and shoulder area, freeing the brachial plexus so you are fully prepared for the complete inversion in Shoulderstand Vinyasa.

The Bridge pose is very beneficial for strengthening the buttock muscles, hamstrings and lower back region, so it is an excellent posture for most back conditions. Likewise it is ideal for practice during pregnancy to maintain strength and alignment of the lower back preventing the occurrence of lordosis (sway back) common during the later phases of pregnancy. It is also beneficial for people with sciatica (inflammation of the sciatic nerve), characterized by shooting pains down the back of the hip and/or leg.

This pose with personally adapted variations is used frequently for such conditions as prolapse of the uterus and colon, gastritis, colitis, sciatica, as well as hernia and knee strains – either upon the patellar ligament, the cartilage (medial meniscus), or the ligaments of the knee joint.

The Bridge pose is also beneficial for strengthening the heart, as blood supply is increased to the heart during the pose, and thus challenges the heart muscle in a way that is not strenuous. The effect can be progressively increased so that the heart muscle is strengthened over time. It has many of the same benefits as the Shoulderstand in that blood supply is increased to the neck and head region as well, but can be safely practiced by people who have neck injuries, or by diabetics.

The sequence concludes with a twisting pose called the Abdominal Twist, Jathara Parivartanasana, which complements the motions of the Bridge pose by giving a rotation to the hips and abdominal area. The Abdominal Twist is an excellent pose for stretching and toning the lateral muscles of the hips and thighs. A manipulated version of this pose is used commonly by chiropractors to adjust a large area of the spine ranging from the sacral to the mid thoracic area. Thus it is not uncommon to experience spontaneous "chiropractic adjustments" during the practice of this twist. The snapping and popping of joints which sometimes occurs in this posture and in other twists should not be encouraged, but rather just be allowed to happen. By lengthening the spine as you twist, the incidence of cracking sounds will lessen. Frequent cracking of the spinal joints may cause a weakness of the joint capsule or the deeper layers of the erector spinae muscles. Avoid adjusting your spine with regular chiropractic treatments as the spine can become unstable rather than strong in alignment. Once a month should be the maximum except for care to an injury.

The realignment of the lower spine can be performed more specifically, more correctly, with the help of a trained Structural Yoga Therapist or a bodyworker familiar with yoga practices. As your muscles become freed, the ligaments holding the vertebrae are also loosened, and postural distortions can be corrected to some extent. If your goal includes postural improvement and vertebral alignment, I recommend you seek out a certified Structural Yoga Therapist as listed on my website.

The natural curves of the spinal column should be maintained in all postures so that strength is encouraged; whereas when the spine is lax and loose adjustments and snapping are much more common. In Yoga our aim is to strengthen the spine and maintain natural spinal curves, and if realignment is necessary, it can be a secondary aspect of the work. More of our concern in Yoga is toward strengthening the mind as an energy body. Sometimes realigning the physical body is helpful in providing this energy upliftment in the subtler body.

The final pose of the sequence Apanasana, or Energy Freeing pose, is beneficial for relieving pressure in the lower abdomen and back. Here it serves as a counterpose to the backbending of the Bridge pose variations. It is ideal to practice this asana dynamically, going into and partially out of the pose repetitively, when there is a strain or injury to the lower back. After this dynamic method has been done with no side affects, then the pose can be done statically – five to ten minutes or more is not an uncommon recommendation for people with strain in the lower back section. The posture creates strength in the deeper muscles of the abdominal region and the hip flexors, including the iliopsoas. These muscles are very important in maintaining strength and alignment of the lower spine, so Apanasana should be held for at least six breaths or longer.

Apana is one of the five functions of Prana. When Apana is active it propels waste material out from the pelvic cavity. This prana is the propellant force behind urination, menstruation, and defecation. When it is in harmony the menstrual cycle is regular and comfortable. Holding the pose with prolonged exhalation and focusing upon relaxing the lower abdomen will help to stabilize this subtle biological energy pattern.

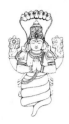

Bridge Vinyasa
Setubandhasana
Mukunda Stiles © 2007

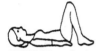 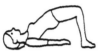 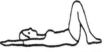 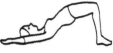

1- EXHALE knees bent with feet/knees 6" apart.

2- INHALE, raise hips. Bridge Pose.

3- EXHALE down. AFTER EXHALE arms over head on floor.

4- INHALE, raise hips.

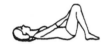 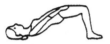 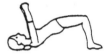

5- EXHALE, down. AFTER EXHALE hands on thighs shoulders rounded

6- INHALE raise hips.

7- EXHALE down. AFTER EXHALE form outward fingerlock.

8- INHALE raise hips.

  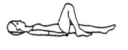 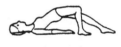

9- EXHALE down. After EXHALE arms shoulder level.

10- INHALE raise hips.

11- EXHALE down. After EXHALE hands beside hips, left leg straight.

12- INHALE raise hips level. EXHALE down. Reverse side.

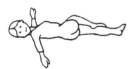 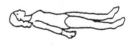

13- After EXHALE, right foot on left knee, arms straight across, twist knee to left. Abdominal Twist - Jathara Parivartanasana. Take 6 full breaths, then reverse.

14- EXHALE, pull knees to chest Energy Freeing Pose - Apanasana

15- INHALE, lower legs. Rest. Corpse Pose - Savasana

Shoulderstand — Sarvangasana Vinyasa

Salamba Sarvangasana

The name for Shoulderstand is literally translated as the "support of the entire body" asana is considered to be the Mother of all the asanas. As an evolved mother nurtures her family and cultivates a healthy society, so this pose is known as the one that cultivates the governing system of the body, the endocrine system. The endocrine glands regulate the physiological functions of the entire body from respiration to hormone secretions to growth patterns and the process of giving life through pregnancy. Shoulderstand is especially regarded for helping thyroid problems. Yet little is understood about its physiology, let alone how inverted postures may help hypo or hyperthyroid conditions. Recent research is still uncovering new insights into fundamentals of the endocrine system and their interactions for wellness. In the same way Yoginis have a lot to learn from being persistent and sattvic in their intimate relations with this "Mother."

Contemplation (Dharana)

The Mother of the Universe

Nicholas Roerich (1874-1947) was a Renaissance man of remarkable talents. He is known as a spiritual artist, philosopher, educator, explorer, archaeologist and especially as a peacemaker. "He left a legacy of 7,000 paintings, drawings, and set designs; thirty books; and countless articles and lectures. The Roerich Peace Pact – a remarkable treaty that sought to preserve cultural monuments during time of war – signed in the White House in the presence of President Roosevelt and other world leaders, earned the artist a nomination for the Nobel Peace Prize." [89] "To him the most universal of all the great teachers, the very symbol of spiritual and cultural unity, is the Mother of the World, and he painted this subject many times throughout his career. A veil conceals her eyes, signifying that certain mysteries of the universe are not yet known to man." [90] This is the Mother who has form.

In many traditions the Mother is the Source of Life, depicted both with forms and without. The Buddhist tradition was brought to Tibet from northwestern India by Padmasambhava, the "lotus born" teacher, in the 8th century. He gave the full range of Tantrik transmissions ranging from rituals for cultivating mindfulness to direct realizations of the highest illumination. The only text he composed is the Upadesadarsanamala, A Garland of Profound Advice on The Ways of Seeing Reality. In these Dzogchen (nondual) teachings four goals are spoken of "1) approach – knowing the bodhicitta, the mind of enlightenment; 2) close approach – knowing yourself to be the actual deity; 3) attainment – generating the realization of the Great Mother (Prajnaparamita - perfect wisdom); and 4) Great attainment - the union of method and wisdom.

The Great Mother is the "mother" of all that arises from the infinite sphere of space that which appears as the forms of the four elements of earth, water, fire and air, and all that is able to perform a function. The Great attainment is the union that from the very beginning, conjoins profound emptiness, the space of the mother, and the wisdom of the five great mothers (Buddha consorts) with wishlessness, the aggregates (skandhas that are the father of all Buddhas." [91]

For Yogis the Shoulderstand cultivates the spectrum of awareness that begins as space and manifests as all the elements that comprise the body and the universe. Space is the fifth chakra and residing in this pose brings attention to that element. By inverting the chakra field and imbibing that field of consciousness (literally Viparita Karani Mudra), the Yogini enters into the space of the Great Mother, the Mother of the Universe. The process unveils the form as it reveals the formless Mother to be beyond the "perfect wisdom" of Prajnaparamita, beyond Her other forms, generating an awareness of wisdom (4th kosha) that extends beyond the known revealing what hidden mysteries She is ready to reveal. The pose is only for health of the body; but the mudra is for the propagation of Spiritual illuminations.

Precautions –

Anyone with chronic concerns in the following areas is well advised to seek the supervision of a competent Yoga Therapist so that practice can be adapted to suit you.

<u>Low back injury:</u>

Do not practice this Vinyasa without your teacher closely watching. Work with the individual components of the Bridge Vinyasa first before doing the entire series. The prerequisite to doing the flow is to do all variations of the Bridge pose until they can be comfortably held for six breaths. Then, work with the Shoulderstand Vinyasa gently, extending yourself gradually into each position. Avoid doing the poses to your full range of motion.

<u>Neck and upper back injury:</u>

Do not attempt the Shoulderstand or Plow poses until you can perform both of the Preparatory exercises for twelve repetitions each. This will build the necessary strength in the upper back and shoulder muscles so you will bear your body's weight on your shoulders and not on your neck during all the poses including the full Shoulderstand.

<u>Women during the menstrual flow:</u>

It is recommended that you do not do any inverted poses the first three days of the cycle, or while your flow is heavy. The Shoulderstand helps the body absorb nutrients from the small intestine as it inverts the organs, thus it increases Udana and Samana Prana. As menstruation is a time of release and purification, Apana Prana is increased at that time. Thus because of these opposing pranic processes, Shoulderstand should not be done during menstrual flow.

<u>Diabetics and those with concerns for detached retinas:</u>
Do not do any inversions or forward bends where your head is lower than your heart, as they may cause irreparable damage to your retina.

Preparatory Exercises

Cat Bow - Marjarasana

This movement came from Kali Rae of Tri Yoga International. I find it is of tremendous benefit in situations where weak arms and shoulders would otherwise contribute to pain.

Begin on your hands and knees, hands shoulder width apart, fingers pointing straight ahead. INHALE arch spine downward in cat lift phase, as in the image on the left.

EXHALE bend the elbows, lowering the chest halfway toward the floor moving forward as you come downward. Keep the head up with your neck long, shoulders pulled back and down with your elbows close to your sides. Cat bow is the image on the right.

After the test INHALE return to straight arm phase. To develop strength do the motions in rhythm with your breath exhaling down and inhaling up. Over time increase your repetitions to twelve which is the minimum prerequisite for a safe Shoulderstand.

This exercise enhances the natural curve of the cervical region and strengthens the supportive muscles of the neck and head. It also develops strength in the back of the shoulders (triceps, trapezius, latissimus and posterior deltoid), lessening the tendency for rounded shoulders and poor posture.

Neck Strengthening

1 - Lie on your back with knees bent, feet close to hips. Place your hands be side your head with the elbows at a right angle straight opposite your shoulders, as shown above. Draw your shoulder blades together and down toward the pelvis to keep the upper and middle trapezius muscle engaged. This will isolate the neck muscles from the shoulder muscles, to fully tone your neck.

2 - EXHALE and lift your head up tucking the chin down toward the collarbone. INHALE as you lower your head. Relax all facial and neck muscles completely before you repeat. Repeat the motion. Stop when you feel fatigue or shaking. Optimal strength is twelve repetitions.

3 - Next turn your head to the left. While keeping the arms on the floor, lift the head watching the left elbow. INHALE as you lower the head. Optimal strength is six repetitions. Reverse for the right side.

4 - When the optimal level is reached, then you may perform a series that combines all the motions. EXHALING while lifting the head to center. Then keeping the head lifted, rotate to the right looking at the elbow, then again to center. Then to the left, back to center and lower slowly while gazing down at the breastbone.

This exercise isolates the sternocleidomastoid muscles located on either side of the neck. These neck muscles rotate the head and flex the neck to look down. They are commonly weak due to the stress and tightness that accumulates in their neighboring muscle, the trapezius, which runs like a shawl across the neck, shoulders and upper back. This exercise is of great benefit for chiropractic patients, often eliminating frequent neck adjustments.

Shoulderstand Vinyasa Instructions –

1. Begin by lying on your back, knees up, feet resting on the floor hip width apart. Rest your arms at your sides with your palms upward.
2. INHALE as you lift your hips from the floor raising yourself into the Bridge pose. EXHALE and hold for 3 breaths, then
3. INHALE clasp your hands behind your back to squeeze your shoulder blades. Then separate your hands to outwardly rotate your shoulders with palms upward fully expanding your chest so that your weight is on the upper outer arms. Stay for three breaths.
4. EXHALE relaxing your shoulders as you lower your hips, returning to the starting position.
5. INHALE bend knees to chest, then raise your legs straight up to form an "L" in the Upward Extended Leg Pose (Urdhva Prasarita Padasana). Stay for three breaths.
6. EXHALE into Energy Freeing pose (Apanasana) pulling your thighs toward your ribcage while pressing your hands onto the floor. INHALE then firmly push the floor as you
7. EXHALE to roll your hips up so that your legs become parallel to the floor.
8. INHALE as you clasp your hands and draw your shoulder blades together to expand your chest. Come onto the outer top of your arms. EXHALE and continue to adjust until you are Satisfied bearing your weight on your shoulders in the Half Plow pose (Ardha Halasana).
9. INHALE and lower your hips to the support of your hands at the pelvic rim (iliac crest). Keep your legs straight, raising them to a 45-60 degree angle from the floor. Adjust yourself for stability then remain steady for six breaths in Inverted Action (Viparita Karani Mudra).
10. INHALE and press your back ribs upward and forward to extend yourself into the full Supported Shoulderstand (Salamba Sarvangasana). Hold only if you are comfortable.
11. EXHALE lowering your straightened legs to the floor over your head while lowering your arms behind your back in a relaxed Plow position (Halasana). INHALE to lift your chest so that your spine does not press the floor. Stay for three breaths.
12. EXHALE and lower your hips coming back into the Inverted Action position. Stay for six breaths with your back in a relaxed position.

13. EXHALE lowering your arms palm down, then firmly press the floor to slowly roll your back down. Rest with your legs extended straight up, returning to the Upward Extended Leg pose. Then INHALE as you lower your legs to the floor in one continuous breath.

14. EXHALE placing your hands beneath your hips or thighs. Then INHALE fully lifting your chest, tilting your head back to gently rest on the crown of your head. Remove and replace arms so that your shoulders move back and down allowing you to be supported by your shoulder muscles. This is the Fish pose (Matsyasana). Stay in the pose for at least twelve slow, complete breaths. Keep tilting your pelvis backward to tense your abdominals, yet maintain your lumbar curve. INHALE deeply pushing your elbows into the floor to take pressure off your head. Then EXHALE tilting your pelvis backward to roll your spine down to the floor from lower to upper back so the head is the last to come to the floor.

15. Open your legs and arms to a comfortable position and rest in Corpse pose. (Savasana). Breath deeply encouraging relaxation and opening yourself to the full benefits of the Vinyasa.

Notes to polish your practice –

The main consideration I have with this series is to protect your neck and shoulders by thoroughly preparing for the sequence. Once you are fully developed in these preliminaries and the Bridge Vinyasa is consistently comfortable, then you are ready for this Vinyasa.

Many teachers encourage the use of a host of props for the Shoulderstand. I find they are unnecessary for students who are assessed by their ability to use the proper muscles in all the preliminary practices. If is only a lack of sequential development of tone that brings about a need for props.

Benefits –

The Shoulderstand has been called the Mother of all the asanas: "As a mother strives for harmony and happiness in the home, so this asana strives for harmony and happiness of the human system."[92]

The Shoulderstand Vinyasa is a very powerful sequence of poses that invert the body and reverse the normal gravitational influence upon circulation. This especially increases the flow of blood to the head and neck. Initially there is a decrease in blood pressure and with a prolonged stay an increase in blood pressure. There are many benefits to this reversal. Among them is the reverse of gravity upon the digestive organs. Also the Classical Yoga texts cite the reverse of the Sun and the Moon energies of the belly and third eye, respectively, as enhancing spiritual awareness.

For people without back or neck problems, the Shoulderstand Vinyasa is ideal for relieving the pressures and strains of the day, relieving tension in the shoulder muscles. The inversion often stimulates peristalsis in the intestines for more complete digestion.

The Shoulderstand position, Salamba Sarvangasana, in which the body is in an erect position, is equally beneficial to the half position known as Viparita Karani Mudra. Mudras tend to induce the feeling of sensory withdrawal, pratyahara, the fifth step of Classical Yoga. When mastered the mudra will greatly help deepen pranayama and meditation practices. The physical practice of Inverted Action brings the weight of the body onto the back of the upper arms, thus building strength in the biceps and triceps muscles.

In the plow posture the spinal stretch is increased squeezing the blood flow into the neck and head areas in a deeper manner than with the Shoulderstand. The lift of the torso is achieved by the strength of the mid back (trapezius and latissimus), thus the weight should be taken by the shoulders and not by the back.

The beginner should practice the Fish pose for a short period, but once they learn to adjust their effort level to sustain comfort, the duration should be lengthened. According to my first teacher, the Fish should be held for half the total time spent in all the inverted poses. In this manner it reverses the cervical flexion of the Shoulderstand and opens the baroreceptorbarroreceptor reflex of the neck that restores blood pressure to normal.

In the Fish posture the spine is reversed in a full backbend (with cervical extension) increasing blood flow into the neck and head areas in a reversal of the Shoulderstand placement where the neck is in flexion. This is a remarkable posture, in that once perfected, the practitioner can do the pose in water, lifting the chest upward such that the body can float for an extended period of time without any movement of the limbs. The buoyancy comes from filling the upper lungs completely and keeping the chest fully expanded. It is done with the legs together, the hands behind the low back to assist in lifting the chest, so that only the face and upper chest is out of the water. When done in this way, you can remain afloat for some time, depending upon your ability to relax in this floating position.

Together these poses especially relieve the most common area of tension in the body, the trapezius muscle, which runs across the upper back extending up the neck to the base of the skull. The word trapezius comes from the Greek word for shawl. The muscle is shaped in a down pointing triangle, like a shawl when draped over the shoulders.

The final posture, the Corpse pose, should be held for a longer stay than normal, with the limbs separated further from the torso than usual to allow maximum circulation benefits.

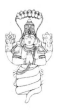

Shoulderstand Vinyasa
Salamba Sarvangasana
Mukunda Stiles © 2007

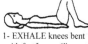

1- EXHALE knees bent
with feet/knees 6" apart

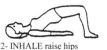

2- INHALE raise hips
Bridge - Setubandhasana
EXHALE hold pose, 3 breaths

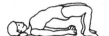

3- INHALE join hands to
squeeze scapula then
separate them, rolling
shoulders outward

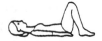

4- EXHALE lower hips

5- INHALE, legs up
Upward Extended
Leg Pose - Urdhva
Prasarita Padottanasana

6- EXHALE knees to chest
INHALE then strongly
push the floor as you

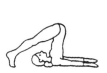

7- EXHALE raise legs parallel
to floor.

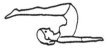

8- INHALE, interlace fingers
& pull back straight. Half Plow
Ardha Halasana.   EXHALE

9- INHALE support pelvis
raising legs to Inverted
Action - Viparita Karani Mudra
Relax your effort for 3 breaths

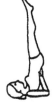

10- INHALE straighten
body to Supported
Shoulderstand Pose
Salamba Sarvangasana
Hold if comfortable

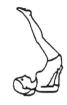

11- EXHALE lower legs to
Plow Pose - Halasana
stay for 3 breaths

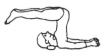

12- INHALE return to
Inverted Action Mudra
stay for 3 breaths

13- EXHALE lower back
Upward Extended Leg Pose
INHALE lower legs

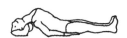

14- EXHALE hands under thighs
INHALE chest up, head on floor
in Fish Pose - Matsyasana
3 breaths

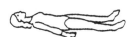

15- RELAX opening legs and
back to Corpse Pose -
Savasana

XII. Ayurvedic Yoga Therapy

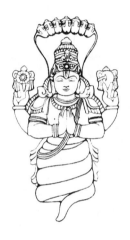

Ayurvedic Yoga Therapy incorporates all three styles of doing Yogasanas, as the teachings are custom designed according to the student's Ayurvedic constitution, health, sex, age, temperament, interest, and spiritual inclination. According to the great yoga master Professor Shri T. Krishnamacharya – teacher of world-renowned Yogis Pattabhi Jois, BKS Iyengar (his brother-in-law), TKV Desikachar (his son and successor) and Indra Devi (the first woman of Yoga) – the secret of yoga is to adapt yoga to the individual. I have written about the physical nuances that teachers and individuals need to consider in using this principle to help themselves or their students receive the maximum structural benefit from Yoga asanas.[93] His methodology is best suited for individual presentation, not in a class format where the individuals must learn to make themselves fit the style that is being presented.

In many class situations, the individual may be mismatched in terms of their Ayurvedic constitution to the constitution of the Yoga being practiced. Typically, Yoga is not adapted to their changing cycle of life or health, but rather the individual is learning to adapt themselves to the Yoga taught. This does not suit either the classical teachings of Ayurveda or of Yoga. By knowing the Ayurvedic make-up, the Classical Yoga Teacher or Therapist can prescribe not only the school of Yoga suitable to the student but also personalized practices within that system for obtaining the optimal benefits from their Yoga sadhana.

There has been a significant amount of literature praising Yoga for its therapeutic benefits. For example "In a nationwide survey of sufferers of virtually every back ailment, Yoga Therapy was shown to provide the most effective form of relief. 93% of those surveyed found Yoga provided dramatic to moderate long-term help. Those who were helped the most got started with professional and personalized instruction."[94] The need for personalized instruction is crucial in making Yoga into a therapeutic modality as well as a spiritual practice that generates enduring serenity.

The scope of conditions to which Yoga Therapy can be applied is widening. This individualized manner of presentation is quite desirable for both health and spiritual evolution. It is in alignment with the classical teachings of Ayurveda and Yoga. By knowing the Ayurvedic imbalance, the Yoga Teacher and/or Ayurvedic Practitioner can prescribe teaching methodology and personalized practice for obtaining the optimal benefit from Yoga sadhanas.

Yoga Practices for Balancing Ayurvedic Doshas

The practice of Yogasanas can imbalance or balance the doshas. When the doshas are balanced, the result automatically takes the Yogi through the sequence of experiences described in the <u>Yoga Sutras</u>. By paying attention to the doshic qualities during practice, one can more readily allow the inward state of mind necessary for maintaining an awareness of your true Self.

Our constitution depends on the configuration of doshas; they influence our body structure and function as well as our emotional and psychological reactions. As external conditions change, for example time of day or weather, changes in diet might be necessary to maintain balanced health. Different Yoga poses as well as different methods to do familiar poses may also be used to regulate internal changes and provide balance to the doshas and the gunas.

Asanas can be classified according to the dosha they balance. Many postures inherently push on the seat/home of the doshas, although practices that are balancing to the individual doshas are those that are characterized by as many doshic attributes as possible. The seat of Vata is the pelvic cavity and colon organ, sitting poses have the ability to stimulate or balance Vata dosha. The seat of Pitta is the abdominal cavity and the small intestine, thus twisting and backbending poses whose major affect is on the abdomen and middle back can affect Pitta dosha. The seat of Kapha is the chest and the stomach; poses like Bridge (Setubandhasana) and Shoulderstand (Sarvangasana) can affect Kapha dosha.

More important even than where yogasanas work in your anatomy is how they are practiced. Second, one's constitution will determine the manner in which one approaches their sadhana practices. A balanced Vata predominant student would seek a long-term practice that emphasized relaxation and spirituality that could be studied for a lifetime; while an unbalanced Vata would tend to jump from one method to another, seeking to solve their current problems or stress and then moving on to something more in vogue. In this pattern they will tend to forget about the benefits they had received and loose any insights into the efficacy of the practice.

A balanced Pitta predominant student would seek a practice that is stimulating and has enough variety to keep them from getting bored; however, an unbalanced Pitta would do this practice intensely until a repetitive motion injury or inflammation developed, then switch to another activity altogether, like rollerblading.

A balanced Kapha predominant student would seek a method that appeals to their sensitive and devotional nature, while also challenging to their desire for physical fitness. An unbalanced Kapha would come for Yoga class to loose weight but would stop if they became tired or depressed.

Classical Yoga following Ayurvedic guidelines can be presented in a class format, adapting the practices according to the changes in season and when the class is small enough, to the individual temperaments of committed students. For instance, Vata harmonizing practices during the spring and fall when weather is changeable; in this way, the yoga students can adapt to their own internal and external changes. Kapha balancing practices would be given during the winter months to help one adapt to the cold and can help with issues of attachment or detachment. These Kapha practices will also promote stamina, strength, and enhance the immune system. Pitta balancing practices will be given in the summer to help us adapt to the heat of summer and also strengthen the Agni, improve circulation and restore discrimination to critical or frustrated mental states.

A mixed dosha format can be used within the Classical Yoga format. The optimal sequence for a full practice is to first gently balance Vata, then Pitta, then Kapha and ending by taking Vata's pranic energies into a deeper more meditative state. The Vata Yoga practice consists mainly of specific gentle vinyasas performed rhythmically with harmonious ujjaye pranayama and learning how to retain the increased prana. The Pitta Yoga presentation emphasizes a moderately aerobic method of practice with focus upon stretching the muscle tissue and generating the internal heat of tejas. Kapha Yoga encourages stamina, holding of the postures with a devotional attitude to elevate Kapha thus stimulating the production of ojas. The natural result of a thorough Classical Yoga sadhana is for the doshas to be elevated from the grosser elements to the subtler qualities as prana, tejas and ojas.

Regulating Yoga Practices

The optimal Yoga program will incorporate three considerations. Practices for maintenance of health, therapeutics for the removal of dis-eases, and for spiritual development. A program that is imbalanced will tend to generate problems in the various dimensions.

The interaction of Yoga and Ayurveda for the reversal of specific conditions is first mentioned in the Hatha Yoga Pradipika.

"One who practices Yoga erroneously, contracts diseases of Vata."
HathapradipikaV, 1. [95]

Svatmarama Yogi, the author of this 14th century manuscript, believed that disease-producing obstruction could be removed and the natural functioning of Prana could be restored by slowing and deepening the breath and directing the Prana to painful parts of the body. For details on this process see sutras 9 - 11. Therapies related to Vata are of prime interest, and within this scope, the proper movement of Prana is foremost. "According to ancient Indian pathology, every disease by necessity involves Vata dosha. There are no purely Pitta or purely Kapha diseases though there may be a purely Vata disease." [96] To comprehend the path of Prana as it courses through the various bodily channels, is to be able to see the formative qualities affecting all the dimensions (koshas) of the Yoga student, as well as the consciousness that generates spiritual or mundane virtues.

The research into and the applications of Yoga Therapy for pathological conditions is as varied as the diverse approaches to Yoga practice. The different approaches also differ in their recommendations for various conditions.   Dr. S. L. Vinekar, former director of the famous Kaivalyadhama Yoga Institute near Poona, India, made a summary of the practical application of Yoga Therapy. This was the first center for the scientific study of Yoga, conducting research since 1926 published in its quarter pamphlet, Yoga Mimamsa. "The Yogic Therapy as such cannot be of much use in acute diseases nor in infective processes, but it can prevent such attacks by improving one's general resistance and power of immunity. It could also provide rehabilitation after the diseases have been tackled successfully, and help restoration of functions that can be called a real cure of diseases. In chronic infective processes, it can provide an efficient ancillary treatment. This will require a good understanding cooperation between the doctor and the Yoga Therapist." [97]

Yoga for Vata

General Considerations

Vata predominant constitutions need a container to hold themselves in balance. The first and most obvious way to create a container is by regulating your lifestyle. Relaxation, pranayama and meditation practices affect the subtler qualities of Vata and if emphasis is placed there first, it can create a grounded personality. A regulated lifestyle that seeks to balance biological rhythms with eating, relaxation, exercise, and working is most important. When this is achieved, the rhythms that are less under conscious control – eliminating, menstruating, and deep sleep - begin to come into harmony. Once a regulated lifestyle is established, then the subtler aspects of Vata can be addressed successfully.

The routine of a Yoga residential or retreat environment can help you to experience the benefits of this rhythm and one can learn how to adapt your life to these principles. This includes arising before dawn and beginning your personal Yoga practice. Breakfast follows, and then work with a break in the middle of the day for a light walk prior to lunch and following it before the afternoon work. Lunch is the optimal time for the heaviest meal of the day. After work is over then time can be best spent unwinding from the day with an early evening Yoga practice. This can be followed with a light dinner such as soup and salad or lunch leftovers. Keeping leftovers over night they will loose their prana, making such food ama (not nurturing, not Mothering, but toxic). Evening is a good time for socializing and sharing of the events of the day with your loved ones. If the day has been challenging then an additional yoga practice composed of restorative poses and/or Yoga Nidra will be rejuvenative prior to meditation and prayer practice. This final Vata balancing practice of the day can even be done lying in bed as you transition to deep sleep.

Over my life, I have experienced the tremendous benefits of a disciplined lifestyle through visits ranging from weekends to half a year at a variety of Yoga and Zen Buddhist residential centers. A wonderful freedom comes from this type of predictable routine. At first one is likely to resist discipline, but over time, its ability to balance Vata and calm excessive thinking becomes clear. There begins to arise a profound relaxation as caretaking of the body and mind tend to lift the veil from the omnipresent Spirit. Once the basics of the daily routine are taken care of spiritual questions such as "where am I going?" can be visited with a gentleness seldom seen elsewhere.

Without this one can lose connection to "right relations" with friends, students, family and even oneself. Maintaining this regular, predictable lifestyle allows life to fall into proper perspective.

Once a regular lifestyle is established, prana will find its home in the pelvic region and the sub pranas will naturally begin to return to their home sites as well. Vata needs attention and seasonal adjustments to maintain its natural ability to balance the changes that are part of life. I typically change my routine every season to adapt to the weather and also to adapt to my current stage of life. This helps to balance the air element as the grosser level of Vata. Once this occurs then the ether element of Vata can be addressed.

The second way to balance Vata is by doing Yoga practices which promote flexibility and sensitivity with specifically sequenced Vinyasa practices. The key is to regulate the breath in a gentle, yet deliberate manner such as with Ujjaye Pranayama. Using this method with the Sun Salutation as the Vinyasa, one cycle will take about 60 seconds. Movement is slow and deliberate with concentration on the internal wave motion and glottal sound of the Ujjaye breathing pattern. The breath leads the motions with the body following its direction.

According to Patanjali,

> Yoga pose
> is a steady
> and comfortable position.
> Yoga pose is mastered
> by relaxation of effort,
> lessening the tendency
> for restless breathing,
> and promoting an identification
> of oneself as living
> within the infinite breath of life.[98]

I placed emphasis on the phrase "yoga pose is mastered by relaxation of effort as it is this quality that brings Vata to balance. Yoga done with Patanjali's guidelines in mind promotes peace, heightens sensitivity, and leads to contemplative insights. This will result to taking actions upon the appropriate revelations. There is a natural evolution of the balanced Vata to stimulate Pitta, increasing the desire to engage in beneficial actions. If practiced regularly, it also releases suppressed fear and curbs anxiety. A sense of attainable aspirations comes into focus and one's burdens are lifted. This practice can also increase the amount of Prana that can be retained to stabilize and balance the five Pranas, and help the mind to stay focused.

My guru, Swami Muktananda said,

> "if the body is weak, prana flows in and out.
> When this is the case, how can you find any joy in life?"

For Vata predominant constitutions – Vata/Pitta, Vata/Kapha, and Vata/Pitta/

Kapha - alertness to the breath and pranic flows within the body can generate an ability to stay balanced longer. The development of prana as a refinement of the breath leads to the highest balance of this element. Breath and body sensations become prana and they stay longer in their appropriate body regions performing their five specific subdosha functions.

The generic prana will gradually reveal its family of sub pranas. Over time when practice is done beautifully, it is possible to experience each of the five subtle pranic movements occurring within their home sites. The pranas are balanced from their grosser forms to the subtlest form as Vyana Prana, resulting in the experience of omnipresence. As Patanjali says,

> In the fourth method
> of regulating one's breath,
> prana is extended
> into the divine life force
> and the range of prana
> is felt permeating everywhere,
> transcending the attention
> given to either
> external or internal objects.[99]

This result arises as a mixture of self-discipline and Grace.

Exercise in General

Vata predominant people need to experience stability and grounding as they engage in exercise that does not fatigue them. Walking with breath timed to be in harmony with the natural swaying of the arms and legs will help to release suppressed emotions and excess thoughts. When this is done in a natural environment free from distractions, Vata will come to balance gently and easily. Even a short walk following meals can help to promote harmony in those of this sensitive constitution.

Yoga Poses

Vata predominant students need to practice poses that focus on the pelvic region and the colon, which are the main sites of Vata. The most useful poses promote freedom in the major joint areas of the lower body– the hips, lumbar spine, and knee joints. Forward bending poses are good, but should not be forced or held in a prolonged fashion. Some Vatas are naturally flexible and must be cautioned not to promote any increased range of motion, which can diminish their prana, their will power and their ability to hear their own inner voice.

Balancing poses such as those in the Balancing Tree Vinyasa - Balancing Tree (Vrksasana), Eagle (Garudasana), and Dancer King (Natarajasana) - will increase concentration. This tends to make Prana smoother, steadier, and when accompanied by Pranayama, refined and subtle.

A Vata balancing practice would place primary emphasis on developing sensitivity through inquiry practices. Asking "what do I feel?" and "where do I feel it?" does more to balance Vata than anything else. The deeper a Vata can go inside, the better.

Asanas should be done with rhythmic, steady and regular breathing (Sama Vritti Ujjaye Pranayama – throat breathing of equal effort and duration) mild and gentle in relative silence. Seated poses, which are traditionally used in breathing and meditation, are also recommended for keeping the hips supple and the pelvic floor mobile and open. Among these practices are easy pose - Sukhasana, half lotus - Ardha Padmasana, adept's pose - Siddhasana, and thunderbolt - Vajrasana. It is good for Vata to discipline their memory by learning sequences that build upon previous weeks training. A teacher can promote Vata balance by making their voice soft, quiet and steady to verbally affirm Patanjali's guidelines. By teaching with contemplation of the classical guidelines of the <u>Yoga Sutras</u>, this generates discipline in a consistent manner. Regular deep relaxation and brief guided meditation throughout a class is very important.

Pranayama

Pranayama is more important for Vata predominant students than for Pittas or Kaphas as it soothes their sensitive nature, which is more prone to disturbances than the other doshas. Ujjaye Pranayama should form the core of the Vata pranayama practice. Variations such as alternate nostril breathing (anuloma Viloma) – also known as purification of the subtle channels (Nadi Shodhana in the <u>Hathayoga Pradipika</u> II, 7-10) are useful in balancing Vata. This can be done in the early morning on an empty stomach for up to five minutes.

Once a consistent practice is established, the next step is to learn Mula Bandha and Aswini Mudra. These practices develop the pelvic floor by strengthening the pubococcyogeal muscles, the bladder, and sex organs. On the subtler level, they can help to refine the Pranas, developing the Apana Prana by prolonging the exhale, and Samana and Vyana Pranas by lengthening the Kumbhakas or breath pause. Variations of these practices are innumerable though I do not recommend Vatas do more variety but instead concentrate on deepening their sensitivity to prana. These practices root out disturbed Vata from its home in the pelvic cavity. With patience and persistence, serenity can come from simply doing Ujjaye pranayama with a mild root lock (Mula Bandha) during exhalations.

Purification (Shatkarmas)

In general, cleansing practices for Vata should be mild and done only for brief periods of time during the early phases of the changeable seasons of fall and spring under supervision. Once they learn the practice their trained pranic sensitivity will reveal when and how much is appropriate in the seasons to follow. Strong purification practices like Vamana Dhouti (intestinal cleansing with water) should be avoided. Milder forms of Shatkarma (6 cleansing actions) can be done daily such as Agnisar Dhouti (purifying the fire), Jala Neti (water snuffing), and Tratak (fixed gazing).

Mantra and Meditation

One meaning of the word mantra is "the sound that protects you." Mantras for Vata can be especially beneficial as Vata rules the mind. By receiving a mantra that affirms your spiritual nature or cultivates the process of inquiry into "Who am I?" can help the student go deeper into their inner world. One example is "so' ham" (I am That), known as a breath mantra as the breath is said to make the sound of this mantra as it goes in and out. By repeating so' ham with the inhalation on the first syllable and the exhalation on the second, the vibratory energy of the sound can be directly felt. With persistence and Grace, the vibration of the mantra may be experienced as the vibration of the body or even the cosmos.

Other mantras are variations on the Shakti mantras that honor the qualities of prosperity and abundance as personified by the Goddess Lakshmi or those of the creative energies personified by the Goddess Sarasvati. Sarasvati is the ruler of the first chakra in the pelvic floor region. Lakshmi is the ruler of the second chakra, located in the bladder region. These mantras are particularly good for dispelling the hidden fears that plague Vata, as they create calmness and serenity.

My guru said repeatedly that for Vata predominant students "the mind is like a dangerous dark alley. You should never go there alone. Take the help of a mantra to protect you."

Sadhana

The ideal yogic spiritual path for Vata is Jnana or Raja Yoga. Whatever method they chose should be coupled with the study of the Yoga Sutras supervised by a competent teacher that they have faith in. If the Raja Yoga tradition is not appealing to them, then scriptural study of their religious heritage is recommended. For instance, a Christian Yoga student could study the Bible, especially the Book of Job and the prophets – Daniel, Psalms, and Revelations; a Jewish Yoga student could study the Torah, and be thoroughly engaged in the practice of daily and seasonal rituals. The most important quality is that spiritual practice includes svadhyaya or self-study aided by reflection on a spiritual text of their preference. Optimal if possible is to have time spent with a spiritual mentor.

Ayurveda Yoga Therapy for Vata Conditions

In yoga's repertoire, we have practices for balancing the Vata qualities within us thus promoting natural biological rhythms like menstruation, elimination, sexual expression, speech, sleep, digestion, physical motions; thereby calming the mind, and elevating our intuition. On the therapeutic level, the practices that restore Vata balance are useful for Vata disturbed conditions such as motion sickness, hypertension, poor circulation, headaches, constipation, hypoglycemia, irregular menstrual rhythms, insomnia and epilepsy. The practices of pranayama and meditation can be adapted to address psychological issues of fear, anxiety, fatigue, self-confidence, improve memory and to develop a stronger will power. Note that specific recommendations should be given to each individual based on personal needs.

Summary
The focus for treatment of Vata is upon promoting relaxation and sensitivity to the inner Self. The method for implementing this is through a combination of practices which bring regular attention to breathing and your pranic life force, by vinyasas done rhythmically led by the natural pace of the breath, and movements which put pressure in your pelvis and legs. Some general examples include gentle warm up series such as the Joint Freeing series (Pavanmuktasana) described in Structural Yoga Therapy harmonized at breath pace, the wave breath (ujjaye pranayama), sitting postures, forward bending postures, and Palm Tree or Balancing Tree Vinyasas.

Yoga for Pitta

General Considerations
The next phase of practice involves a focus to promote vitality, greater energy, and sufficient heat to balance the water/fire quality of Pitta. In contrast to Vata balancing, there is little attention paid to the breath except to allow it to move freely. For Pitta, the pacing will tend to be faster because the emphasis here is on a more vigorous practice to generate body heat and occasional perspiration. The pacing of the asana practice needs to be done in such a manner as to retain the Vata balance, yet warm enough to feel Pitta's heat being retained within the belly. This method redirects frustration, anger, and misguided sexuality, which become transformed into creativity and abundant enthusiasm. The Pitta practices will create vitality and luster. It will also increase Tejas, which in its highest form manifests as spiritual discrimination and allows the yogi to see through the ephemeral into the transcendental nature of life.

For Pitta predominant constitutions - Pitta/Vata and Pitta/Kapha - attention directed toward the sensations of heat and vitality are crucial. Once heat is generated and brought home to the belly, the student can learn to discern the five specific subdoshas of Pitta and seek guidance from them. In this manner, Pitta evolves into Tejas.

The yoga practices for balancing Pitta energy promote a good appetite with strong digestive fire, heighten enjoyment of life, and maintain the stability of our vitality. Therapeutically, these practices are used for inflammatory conditions such as arthritis, ulcer, colitis, acne and sciatica. The psychological applications include becoming free from anger, criticism, judgment, dissatisfaction with life and jealousy.

Pittas need practices that are stimulating enough to capture their natural need for excitement. Yet the practice should not stimulate competitiveness or over heat them. The need is for warmth and enthusiasm not a burning heat. Kundalini Yoga is not recommended for this dosha, except under close supervision and while living with other practitioners. Taking plenty of water before and after Yoga is highly recommended.

Exercise in General

The Pitta quality is enhanced by cooperation and sharing activities. Pitta quality will especially enjoy partner yoga practices done in a light hearted jovial manner. Pitta predominant people need this more than others. Working out together and going to Yoga class is more important for them than for Vata predominant people who may tend to be loners.

Yoga Poses

Pitta needs yogic practices that maintain their digestive fire and warm personality, yet temper their tendency toward inflammatory conditions. Yoga poses that apply pressure to the navel region and the solar plexus are beneficial because they provide a massage to the area of the liver and spleen. Spinal twists should be practiced with abdominal focused breathing. Pittas can train themselves to observe the heating tendency of these poses and allow the heat to spread over the skin during winter, thus promoting Bhrajaka Pitta. During the summer, the result should restore the Agni to its home in the middle abdomen, balancing Pachaka Pitta.

Backbending poses, including Cobra (Bhujangasana), Bow (Dhanurasana) and Locust (Salabhasana), stimulate Pitta when it is deficient or sluggish. These should be practiced in moderation or by going in and out of the poses with mild exertion. Holding of these poses is only recommended for Kapha as they can break up the stagnancy and attachment associated with this doshas excesses.

Full headstand should be avoided for more than one minute, as it increases Sadhaka and Alochaka Pitta, which may result in burning eyes or headache. It should be avoided entirely for those persons experiencing spontaneous Kundalini experiences as signs of spiritual or psychic awakenings. Brief handstands are also encouraged.

Milder poses such as Inverted Action (Viparita Karani Mudra), Shoulderstand (Salamba Sarvangasana) and Plow (Halasana) are beneficial in restoring serenity to Pittas when their lifestyle has been too demanding. The classic Hatha Yoga texts Siva Samhita and Gheranda Samhita (see Appendix) speak metaphorically about the balancing of the solar and lunar principles in the human body. In these poses, the moon (cooling) principle in the soft palate region is restored from its tendency to gain heat by dropping its secretions into the navel (sun or heating) center. The net result of good practice is that these poses cool the mind and body. One must adapt the practice daily in terms of effort, duration and focus of breath to restore the fire element to its capacity to produce lightness in the mind.

Pranayama

When the body/mind becomes too hot, Pittas should practice a cooling type of pranayama called Sitali Pranayama. You will find it described in the pranayama section; this is an ideal form for Pitta and can be practiced during the hot period of the year.

In general, Pittas need to practice steadiness with regard to pacing of all Pranayamas, as speeding up will tend to be aggravating. While a moderate practice of Bhastrika may be of benefit during winter, they should avoid an excessive practice that displaced the digestive fire.

Purification (Shatkarmas)

Agnisar Dhouti is an ideal practice for Pitta as it helps to maintain the digestive fire of metabolism (Agni). It can be safely continued for a long period of time, if discernment is maintained to avoid excessive heat or enthusiasm. Nauli is also beneficial for Pittas especially when effort is made to learn the variations of left, right, central and rolling from side to side. For moderate to slender body types this is not difficult to master, though one needs experienced guidance to show the steps to mastering Nauli.

Tratak practice is especially beneficial for Alochaka Pitta. It should be practiced regularly to the point of making the eyes tear. Once this has been achieved, it can be continued until the tears become cool. In those with eyestrain or who wear glasses, Alochaka Pitta may be excessive; this practice will return it to normal levels.

Mantra and Meditation

Pitta will benefit from practicing soothing mantras like Om or the Bija mantras like lam (focusing upon the first chakra) and ram (focusing upon the third chakra). These mantras have a calming affect and help Pittas to experience fire in its spiritual essence as Divine Light.

Many Pitta predominant students meditate more deeply with open eye practices than closed. In this manner the practice of fixed gazing (Tratak) can be evolved into its deeper form as Shambhavi Mudra. This enhances a feeling of serenity, allowing meditation to move towards an experience of selfless service in honor of the Divine Presence in others. It is important for Pittas to maintain humility and selfless service is a key to that quality's evolution. These practices may utilize the aid of a Yantra (spiritual geometric design), by holding their visual awareness still and contemplating the archetypical quality the Yantra represents, thus meditative absorption is deepened, which can focus attention to the subtler body of energy and light. This is particularly recommended for those students of Tantra Yoga.

Sadhana

The deal spiritual practice for Pitta is selfless service (Karma Yoga). Regular readings from the Bhagavad Gita, Paramahansa Yogananda's Autobiography of a Yogi, or the Book of Job in the Bible can provide inspiration. These writings will enhance Pittas understanding of detachment and sense of self.

Another path well suited for Pitta is Tantra Yoga. The deepest aspects of Tantra are transformative, honoring the world as the creation of the Divine Mother. [100] Tantrik teachings that focus upon the more superficial goals of heightened sensuality, heightened sexuality, opening the chakras and psychic abilities will not satisfy Pitta's longing for Spirit.   "Recent Western nonacademic interest in the Tantra has tended to blur the important distinction between the tantra-sastra and the kama-sastra. India had a highly developed science of erotica, the kama sastra, where the goal was a cultured, refined lovemaking, a perfectly acceptable fulfillment of one of the four legitimate aims of human existence, that of kama (sensual pleasure). The Tantra sastra, in using the secret ritual, did not seek to fulfill Kama, but rather to provide a new path for the attainment of moksha (spiritual liberation). . . It grossly distorts the Tantra to represent it as teaching that sexuality and spirituality are themselves identical."[101]

The Yoga Sutras (III, 38) caution about the development of supernatural powers that can result from realizing the potential of the mind. In the third chapter on siddhis, it states: "These gifts (that come from siddhis) are impediments to being absorbed in Spirit, but they are seen as the attainment of perfect to the worldly minded." [102]

Ayurvedic Yoga Therapy for Pitta

In yoga's repertoire we have practices for balancing the Pitta qualities thus promoting natural biological functions of digestive assimilation, eye sight, skin, liver function, and increasing mental property of discernment. On the therapeutic level the practices that restore Pitta balance will diminish Pitta aggravated symptoms such as inflammation, poor circulation, headaches, and strong cramps at the onset of menstrual rhythms. The practices of pranayama and meditation can be adapted to address psychological issues of anger, criticism, self confidence, desire and manifestation of wealth, improve memory, and to develop a persistent will power.

Summary

The focus for treating Pitta is upon maintaining good energy levels through discrimination about what is beneficial and activities which bring out their innate love of life and enthusiastic vitality. Yoga practices are done with occasional attention to breathing, with the main focus upon locating the specific places feeling a stretch, yoga poses vigorously performed, and movements which put pressure in the abdominal cavity. Some specific yoga practices for balancing Pitta include the Sun Salute, Sunbird and Cobra Vinyasas, twists and challenging standing poses such as Triangle and the Warrior.

Yoga for Kapha

General Considerations –

Yoga for Kapha dosha promotes strength, purifies the physical body, and develops stamina, which balances the earth/water quality of Kapha. Attention is focused upon the development of muscle strength and stamina by holding postures within specific Vinyasa sequences. This practice has a grounding benefit. At the same time as one develops strength, one must also soften that strength much as earth is softened by water. This allows the muscles to become strong and defined but not hard and the skin to be soft and malleable. A rock hard physique with too little body fat is the result of overemphasis upon Pitta's fire, which burns away the watery qualities of permeability and openness.

The yogi's body, while not slender and hard contains all the elements, enveloped in a soft warm skin. Swami Prakashananda is one example. His body was round and soft, similar to the body of a woman entering her second trimester of pregnancy. I had seen this in our guru's body and in his guru's body as well. Prakashananda invited me to massage him at the end of each day. I began with his feet, only to find his skin was remarkably soft, luxurious like cashmere, yet also uniquely warm and luminous. I thought it more a pleasure to me than I imagined it might be to him. As I continued up his body, his legs felt majestically strong, yet soft, like redwoods covered in moss. When I reached his belly, I discovered the most unusual sensation of all. His belly jiggled not unlike the "bowl full of jelly" image used to describe Santa Claus. Yet there was another attribute that I could not discern. When I closed my eyes to focus on the tactile sensations, I discovered a vast vision of blue undulating waves of light that resembled the sight of moonlight upon ocean waves. The water element of his body was fully apparent. I had always been told that our body is composed of 70% seawater and here I was experiencing it directly in his yogic body. I have never forgotten this profound revelation.

The amount of time taken to practice a Kapha sequence is longer than for Pitta or Vata. Elongation of the body is promoted by the strength to lift upward against the force of gravity bringing attention to Kapha's home in the chest region. However, a sturdy physique is created not from stretching, but from toning. This level of practice also develops the cardiological and immune systems. Kapha's balance is apparent in very healthy individuals.

By following Patanjali's guides with this practice, the chest is softened as Kapha is sent to its root home in the chest cavity, which opens and softens the heart. The exhale should be longer than the inhale and occasionally the breath should be released through the mouth with am audible sigh. This will help to open hidden, repressed emotions and to release sadness, lethargy, and attachments to unfulfilled desires, while promoting courage, hopefulness, faithfulness and humility. Ultimately, it will increase Ojas. On the physical level Ojas represents health and the strength of the immune system; on the spiritual level, it is imbibing the love of God/dess generating the capacity to love and accept all as Divine. A spiritual practice often becomes central to an evolving Kapha.

For Kapha predominant constitutions – Kapha/Vata and Kapha/Pitta – the primary focus is on purifying the body of excess mucous and weight, so that health is maintained. The deeper level of Kapha practice opens the heart and creates connection to their chosen form of Spirit (Ista deVata). From this, Kapha evolves into ojas, producing a luster and glow of spiritual health.

Yoga practices for Kapha strengthen the heart and skeletal muscles, developing good tone, promoting kindness, compassion and open-mindedness. On a therapeutic level, these practices can decrease symptoms of diabetes, asthma and other respiratory conditions, constipation and angina. On a psychotherapeutic level, they are used for depression, attachment, possessiveness, sadness and for periods of mourning the loss of a loved one.

In order to promote optimal balance of the dual nature of Kapha (earth and water), it is crucial to realize that purification is essential for the development of both physical and spiritual virtues. Kapha needs a systemic movement of water to cleanse cellular tissues and remove obstructions. This kind of consistent internal cleansing is more important for Kapha dosha than for the other doshas for whom a spring and/or fall cleaning is adequate.

Kapha balance promotes both strength and stamina as the natural outcome of a healthy immune system. This in turn promotes the development of the subtle tissue called ojas. It is this essence that is the true sign of health, for longevity is born of ojas. My eldest teacher, Indra Devi, possessed a tremendous amount of ojas. A very diminutive woman from Russian Latvia, Indra Devi was nonetheless a powerhouse of energy, love and service to her thousands of worldwide students. I knew her for over 25 years, before her passing in 2002 just three weeks prior to her 103rd birthday. When I met this "First Lady of Yoga," she was 76 and exhibited tremendous gusto, teaching headstand while wearing an Indian sari. Completely uninhibited she tucked the long folds of cloth between her legs and seemed to levitate as she defied gravity. She broke all laws of physics in coming down just as gracefully. Mataji, or beloved mother as she is called, had a way with people; you would assume she had known everyone in the class for years. She was always able to put people at ease and create the feeling of being in one large nurturing Yoga family. Every encounter I had with her, including being at her 100th birthday party was filled with joy and happiness. She exhibited the true signs of ojas in that she lived her motto of "send love and light to everyone."

Exercise in General

Kapha quality needs to establish regular vigorous exercise that is beneficial for the vital organs of the heart and lungs. Kapha as it evolves will also seek the development of spiritual or heart opening practices that generate feelings of love, joy, and connection to community.

Yoga Poses

As Kapha may have sluggish digestion and metabolism when imbalanced, they should perform practices that affect the region of the abdomen to increase digestive fire. The ideal for them is vigorous exercise done with regular discipline. In the yoga regimen, this should include daily practice of Surya Namaskar. For them, the program should be physically challenging done with effort to develop strong arms, chest and upper back. The program should include a minimum of 15 minutes of vigorous practice. They may need to work up to this level of fitness if they have not been maintaining a physical discipline.

Poses that are particularly beneficial for them include Shoulderstand (Sarvangasana), Bridge (Setubandhasana), Lion (Simhasana), Fish (Matsyasana), Peacock (Mayurasana) and Warrior (Virabhadrasana). The poses that press the upper back and chest should be held to their maximum with a focus upon developing muscular strength in the lower trapezius and latissimus dorsi muscles.

Kapha predominant students should hold their Yoga poses longer than Vata or Pitta predominant types. They need to focus their mind and body on actions that purify them and increase stamina. Long stays in postures can promote both a healthy immune system but also open the physical and spiritual heart.

Along with Yoga, they need to exercise throughout the day by walking in nature, working in the garden or swimming. Being in a natural environment is particularly beneficial for Kapha dosha as it helps to maintain their connection with the earth and cycles of nature.

Pranayama

To keep excessive mucous to a minimum, regularly practice Kapalabhati. Heating pranayamas such as Bhastrika and Surya Bhedana are recommended as well. Uddiyana Bandha should be emphasized once they have mastered the basics of pranayama and have a consistent practice. This will help to maintain the strength of the diaphragm and heart muscles.

Purification (Shatkarmas)

All the purification practices were created for the Kapha predominant constitutions. Nauli and Agnisar Dhouti are especially helpful in maintaining the metabolism. Water snuffing (Jala Neti) helps to keep the sinuses and upper respiratory tract open. These practices can also assist in minimizing Kaphas tendency towards allergies and excess mucous formation.

Mantra and Meditation

Mantras that have a devotional connotation are the best for Kapha. Going to group chanting events such as kirtans and bhajans are very uplifting for this heart centered dosha. Once they have challenged and purified their body, their heart is ready to open wide. Safety is an issue that needs to be addressed, for without the feeling of safety and confidence in their teacher and the practices, Kapha will tend to remain guarded.

Sadhana

The main spiritual practice for Kapha is devotional practices of Bhakti Yoga. Both a physical Yoga and a devotional practice are necessary for Kapha, as one without the other may make them suffer. Devotion without physical discipline will make Kapha stagnate, then they are likely to put on excessive weight; physical exercise without devotion is just simply hard work, leaving Kapha feeling dry. The downside for those who are more drawn to spiritual practices than physical Hatha Yoga is that health declines. My spiritual teacher, Swami Prakashananda, claimed, "Every guru has heart conditions, arthritis and diabetes." For us, it makes more sense to be healthy and have some devotion rather than have enormous devotion to others and not pay attention to the rigors of health maintenance.

Ayurveda Yoga Therapy for Kapha

In yoga's repertoire we have practices for balancing the Kapha qualities thus promoting natural biological functions of the heart, cerebrospinal fluid, lubrication of the joints, mucous membrane, respiration, sensual pleasure, and memory. On the therapeutic level the practices that restore balance will diminish Kapha aggravated symptoms such as congestion, colds, asthma, diabetes, bloating during menstruation, and excessive weight gain. The practices of pranayama and meditation can be adapted to address psychological issues of attachment, coldness, spiritual connection to a higher power, improve memory, and to maintain humility to a higher power.

Summary

The focus for treating Kapha is promoting strength and stamina along with cleansing practices to detoxify the system. The practices should be done with regularity and devotion to develop faith and self-confidence. However, they should not be dry and stoic but rather done with joy and laughter. Yoga is done with a focus upon the strengthening effects during the changes of season; the focus is upon purification practices like water snuffing (Jala Neti) and head shining (Kapalabhati). Poses are held with persistence, and emphasis is on postures that press the chest and challenge upper body strength. Examples of Kapha practices include the Pavanmuktasana series variation (described in my Structural Yoga Therapy book) done to develop strength and stamina of each muscular movement; the Isolation Poses, long Sun Salute series, backbending postures such as fish and camel, and sequences such as Stick and Shoulderstand Vinyasas.

Kaphas need to follow their heart more than any of the other doshas. Whatever makes them connect with their laughter, joy and spontaneity is a spiritual path for them. As Joseph Campbell said in giving spiritual advice to his PBS viewers "Follow your bliss." This is excellent advice for our Kapha dosha.

XIII. Progressive Relaxation Exercises & Yoga Nidra

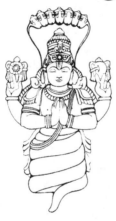

Most students begin a Yoga practice for its well-known benefits to health, vitality and well-being. The Yoga postures are renowned for producing physical fitness and its deep relaxation practices are famous for their dramatic ability to reduce chronic stress. Physical fitness and stress management enhance the functioning of the immune system and produce a radiant glow of well-being.

According to Patanjali's <u>Yoga Sutras</u> II, 47, for the ideal Yoga posture to become perfectly steady and comfortable, one must develop the capacity to direct Selective Relaxation. In good asana practice, you are engaged in directing tension (as muscular exertion) to selective areas of your body, while consciously relaxing the remainder of your body. Through this training, you are encouraged to differentiate between comfortable effort and strain. Taking this further by deepening the relaxation, allows one to discharge even the sympathetic reflexes of tension. For some students, this will release deep-seated fear and other traumatic emotions that the physical body is holing onto. In effective Yoga classes emotional releases are likely to occur, encouraged by both the teacher's and student's comfort with the range of their own emotional expression.

According to Classical Yogic philosophy, stress accumulates in each of the five bodies (koshas). By learning to separate each layer from the others, the Yogini can gain a great degree of self-observation and the detachment necessary to free chronic stress and promote discrimination in becoming liberated from prior conditioning. One complete process for achieving this is known as the Yogic Sleep or Yoga Nidra. This detailed practice has many steps that are designed to be learned over a prolonged period. By taking each dimension sequentially, the Yogini can gain a tremendous freedom from the formative factors of stress.

The first step is to practice the art of physical relaxation. The ideal posture for the practice is the Corpse pose, Savasana. If this is not comfortable, a restorative Yoga posture that facilitates your opening safely can be used. The goal is for you to become absolutely still, eliminating all irregular reflex movements characteristic of stress.

Instructions –
1. Begin in Stick pose, and then bend your knees toward your head, lifting your feet from the floor. Bend your elbows to allow your upper body to round. Then roll your lumbar spine down by using a strong upward thrusting movement of your pubic region as you take your spinal column sequentially onto the floor from the lower to upper region.
2. Once your lower back is flat, rest your upper body weight upon your forearms.
3. Then extend your legs, turning them outward as they open hip width.
4. Reach your arms down and outward from your shoulders to leave your chest lifted and full. This will result in an external shoulder rotation.
5. Tilt your head to look down at your legs, then extend the occipital region at the base of your skull away from your shoulders.

6. Finally, slowly lower your head while maintaining a long naturally curved neckline.

The intention of these instructions is to allow your entire torso; both front and back, to be opened up so that your limbs spread outward and downward from your torso. In this way, all of your joints are comfortably opened. If you are distracted by the position of any limb, by all means continue to adjust yourself to a placement that gives you a sense of physical neutrality. This will show that you are proceeding through the <u>Yoga Sutra</u> guideline and creating a state of detachment. Any tension brings increased body consciousness, yet even this awareness can be utilized to release tension. Whatever adjustments you make should optimize your ability to perceive every part of your anatomy without your attention being forced to be held captive to any part of your body.

By remaining motionless in this position for 10-20 minutes you will automatically be stimulating your "relaxation reflex" originating in your parasympathetic nervous system. No technique is needed except the intention to relax and allow your body to let go of what is no longer beneficial. You will spontaneously begin the process of restoration of your natural stress-free state.

The main goal of this position is to be comfortable enough to have your attention free of your body. If your posture causes physical tension, your mind cannot be focused enough to be directed from one region to another. The most important thing is your comfort and steadiness. Comfort is subjective and cannot be created by conforming yourself to an external "picture perfect" pose. If you are not comfortable and cannot adjust yourself so that relaxation is an automatic event, then ask your instructor for an adjustment. Allow yourself to become limp as they move your limbs or head to provide better support and an opportunity for improved circulation. Allow the adjustments about a minute to take effect. If discomfort persists beyond this point, reposition yourself until you find the optimal placement where your body can surrender to the pull of gravity enough that you feel heavy.

Variation -

If lying on your back is uncomfortable and you are unable to lie still, try lying on your abdomen, feet apart, toes inward and arms folded so that your hands are on the opposite shoulders with your elbows stacked on top of each other. Your nose sits in the fold of your upper elbow to allow your head to be supported while your eyes rest against your biceps. This posture is called the Crocodile (Makarasana), as they have a pointed snout.

If you are pregnant and beyond the first trimester, relaxation can be accomplished by lying on your left side, with knees bent a pillow beneath your head and a second pillow between your knees.

Progressive Relaxation

A number of methods can be used to localize the "relaxation reflex." They can be designed to promote specific parasympathetic reflexes to lower blood pressure, relax a hyperactive colon, or to slow down excessive thinking and help you return to a more responsive state of mind. Relaxation tapes with guided imagery, soothing music, the sounds of nature, a waterfall, etc. are excellent for those whose day has been filled with the tensions of modern living.

For some people going straight into the quiet of relaxation is too abrupt, particularly if you have had continuous overwhelming sensory input. This increases Adya Prana and diminishes the functioning of Samana, Udana and Apana Prana. If your stress levels have been elevated for some time, then I suggest you do the following to gradually release yourself from the layers of cumulative tension. Regular practice of this conscious relaxation using just one or two techniques that are extremely effective will be best.

Yoga Nidra Summary

The process of Yoga Nidra varies according to the amount of time and discipline you wish to create. The full process has 12 stages. [103]

Resolution
Affirmation
Progressive Selective Relaxation
Breath Awareness
Sensory Awareness
Emotional Awareness
Mental Awareness
Imagery
Bliss Awareness
Pure Awareness
Re-Affirmation
Completion

Stage one begins with an attitude that you are going to be attentive and alert through out this process. This involves the use of your will to form a resolution.

Stage two allows you to form an affirmation, to clarify the goal you have for practice.   It is a present tense resolve such as "I am deepening my spiritual life;" or "I am free to uncover my True Self."

Stage three is the process of selective awareness that begins with relaxing the senses associated with the head, starting with the mouth and tongue, lips, face, cheeks, nose, ears, eyes, forehead – right side, left side, third eye; top of the head and back of the head.

Then progressing to the major segments of the body – right side, left side, back, and front.

Stage four focuses on breath awareness and marks the entry into the pranic body. This can be as simple as watching the breath, observing the end points, or adding the breath mantra – ham'sa.

Stage five is sensory awareness - noticing polarities of sensory experience in the present then into the past; cold/hot, moist/dry, pain/pleasure, heaviness/lightness.

Stage six is emotional awareness characterized by the chakras. Here, we feel the poles of our emotional nature – disappointment/contentment, fear/courage, attachment/detachment, sexual arousal/impotence, depression/exhilaration, sadness/happiness, criticism/praise, anger/tolerance.

Stage seven moves us to mental awareness, entering the mind directly. We become aware of current thoughts, then the variety of thoughts that have arisen in the past; pleasant, unpleasant, judgmental, compassionate, lustful, creative, nurturing, destructive.

Stage eight is the use of archetypal imagery to assist our entry into the wisdom kosha. This is the time to use primal images that are universally acknowledged; music, sun, moon, blue sky, Christ, Virgin, guru, cross, or star.

Stage nine moves to the bliss kosha. Experience the joy that arises from your own self, the fullness of your love of all, the joy of being.

Stage ten is pure awareness of the nature of the witness, observing not changing. This is the subtlest sheath, the asmitamayakosha, the witness of "I." It is the eternal sense of self.

Stage eleven is a reaffirmation statement that drives home the affirmation and sets it through all the dimensions of the Self.

Stage twelve is completion; coming back through the koshas to become fully alert and open-eyed.

Take a few breaths with your mouth open on the exhales to release the air that was held in your sinuses, mouth, and trachea passageways. Continue with mouth breathing for three cycles or for as long as you feel tension and fatigue leaving your being. This is the only purpose for which mouth breathing is appropriate. When you feel a sustained reflex of relaxation flowing over your body then gently close your mouth. Continue breathing with a wave pattern flowing downward towards your legs as you inhale. Then feel the flow reversing upward as you exhale while completely relaxing your body.

Let your attention move from point to point through your body, consciously releasing any contractions you discover. If there is tension remaining in your posture, change it at any time. With training, you will develop sensitivity to muscular tension and can eliminate it quickly and effectively by merely a shift of attention. No gross stretch or asana will be needed. Moving to stretch a specific area of tension is less effective for stress management, though for beginners who are kinesthetically oriented, it is necessary until a mental discipline has been secured.

Instructions –

Begin with a resolute intention to stay alert and conscious. The resolution (sankalpa) forms the basis of directing Pitta to balance Vata's pranic currents of sensation. Next rotate your awareness through your body just touching each part with your mind for a couple seconds before moving on to the next part. As you bring each part to awareness, relax it, staying focused on those sensations exclusively.

Begin with an awareness of your right hand thumb (pause), forefinger, middle finger, ring finger, little finger, palm of your hand, wrist, forearm, upper arm, right shoulder, armpit, side of your chest, right side of your waist, right hip, groin, top of your right thigh, knee, shin, ankle, top of your right foot, right great toe, second toe, middle toe, ring toe, little toe (pause). Feel your entire right side (repeat three times, then pause). Remain alert as your feel your right side.

Shift your awareness to your left hand thumb (pause), forefinger, middle finger, ring finger, little finger, palm of your hand, wrist, forearm, upper arm, left shoulder, armpit, side of your chest, left side of your waist, left hip, groin, top of your left thigh, knee, shin, ankle, top of your left foot, left great toe, second toe, middle toe, ring toe, little toe (pause). Feel your entire left side (repeat three times, then pause). Remain alert as your feel your left side.

Bring your attention to the front of your body beginning with an awareness of the top of your right foot, top of your left foot, right ankle, left ankle, right shin, left shin, right kneecap, left kneecap, right thigh, left thigh, genital area, lower abdomen, middle abdomen, upper abdomen, lower ribcage, breastbone, right chest, left chest, front of your neck, lower jaw, chin, lower lip, upper lip, right ear, left ear, right cheek, left cheek, right nostril, left nostril, right eye, left eye, center of your eyes (pause), forehead, scalp, top of your head. Feel the entire front of your body (repeat three times, then pause). Remain alert as your feel your front side.

Bring your attention to the back of your body beginning with the back of your head, back of your neck, right shoulder blade, left shoulder blade, the space between your shoulders, middle back, lower back (pause), right buttock, left buttock, sacrum - the center of your buttocks, back of your right thigh, back of your left thigh, back of your right knee, back of your left knee, right calf, left calf, right heel, left heel, sole of your right foot, sole of your left foot. Feel the entire back of your body (repeat three times, then pause). Remain alert as your feel your back.

Feel your entire body (repeat three times, then pause). Feel every part of yourself. Feel your entire body, whole and complete as your own self (repeat three times, then pause). Remain alert as you feel your entire self. This forms the first stage of the process of Yogic Sleep (Yoga Nidra).

For those who have a more serene lifestyle, a more direct path may work just as well. The only instructions you need are to "simply lay down and relax." I highly recommend that you just go into the position without any mental focus, soothing music, or other stimuli that might become extraneous or distract from focusing upon yourself.

Energy Body Balance

Let yourself settle into the wave pattern of breathing, then scan your body from feet to head. Direct your mind to feel and listen to those sensations, and from the Yogic view of anatomy, result from the subtle energy of Prana. To deepen the relaxation reflex, concentrate on the rising and subsiding energy patterns within your body regardless of where you experience them. As your energy field opens more your awareness of your body's currents of sensation will increase. Allow your body scan to take at least 5 minutes. Remain mentally alert yet physically passive for a minimum of 5-10 minutes after the scan is complete.

When you are complete, roll onto your side and curl up for a few moments of deep breathing before you transition to sitting. Lying on the side tends to put pressure in the armpit stimulating the axillary reflex to open the opposite upper nostril. This reflex is natural and can easily be experienced when the arm is pressed to the ribcage wall. It can also be done seated with a hand pressed into and up against the armpit. This facilitates an opening of the sinuses and clears the mind.

Lying on the left side following Yoga practice is beneficial for stimulating right nostril breathing, which is helpful when you have more activities to do. This is best for morning and early afternoon. Lying on the right side stimulates the left nostril, which is beneficial for stress relief, or as a preparation for sleep. This is the optimal position to lay in bed in as it promotes a deep and prolonged sleep pattern.

Deepening Yogic Sleep to the Other Koshas

You are invited to continue the procedure for up to an hour while directing attention to experiences of the ever-increasing subtler dimensions of yourself. This can progress through your five bodies – physical body structures, subtle body chakras, mind and subtle nerves, intellect and intuitive mind, and finally, the spiritual body that is made of radiant light, the innate life force energy that transcends death. By direct experience one can come to know that innate life force by disengaging from physical, sensory and mental activities. The Yogic Sleep reveals that we are more than who we perceive ourselves to be in our waking state. This procedure has many variations, some of which can arise spontaneously through inquiry into who we are independent of our physiology.

My first exposure to Yoga Nidra came when I was 20 years old. I had been drafted into the army in 1969 during the Vietnam era. Following basic training, I was accepted into West Point Preparatory Academy. The Academy is a one-year school to prepare soldiers on active duty to raise their SAT scores and improve athletic ability to pass the entrance exam to West Point with the highest scores possible.

I had only been there a couple of months when one of my buddies, Bruce Stone, showed me a Yoga book by a student of Ramana Maharshi. I read the introduction and I got the impression that the essence of Yoga was to be able to control your autonomic nervous system. It described how Yogis could control their bodies to such an extent that their breathing could be slowed or stopped and that this could lead to being able to slow or stop your heart. This information peaked my curiosity as I had never considered trying to regulate myself in this manner and I was curious to know what I could do. So we went up into the attic of the barracks to avoid being discovered. There I did the practice described by lying down, concentrating on my breathing and I asked myself to slow it down. It felt natural to slow it until it became suspended. Then, I concentrated on doing the same to my heartbeat. I felt it distinctly and strongly in the middle of my chest, then I concentrated on feeling the rhythm slowing. It complied as easily as had my respiration. Then, my heart beat suspended itself. The first time I tried it I succeeded.

I had stopped my breathing and then my heart. When I did this, I immediately felt myself hovering in the space between the floor and the gables of the roofline. I had gone out of my body. But I had no idea what was happening as I felt myself completely separate from my normal connection with my physical body. My curiosity remained intact though I was startled, not shocked, by the initial experience. I continued to hover near the roof of the building about six feet above Bruce and my body.

The book had not told me of such an event and I did not know how I had gotten here or how to get back into my body. My body was unresponsive to thoughts and I no longer perceived it as myself. There were no sensations emanating from this body into my awareness. I was mystified by the experience. I soon found myself entering a dark place and I began to see four or five beings moving toward me as if back lit by an etheric light had back lighted them. I didn't know who they were or what was happening. My curiosity turned to fear that caused me to become distressed. I began to want to come back to ordinary bodily based consciousness. But I did not know how to transition. How could I communicate to Bruce? He seemed oblivious to the fact that I was no longer in my body. I tried to talk to my body but it was unresponsive to my thoughts. This continued for some time until I heard an extremely serene Voice say, "take a breath."

So I did and suddenly, my mind and body were back in the more familiar environment of being together. I was stunned by the Presence of the benevolent voice I had heard. It was the same voice or Presence I had experienced saving me from a potentially fatal car accident a few months prior to entering the Army.

The experience was totally outside of the red neck world I had been raised in, among the pine forests surrounding majestic Mt. Shasta in far northern California. I had entered another dimension that I now would call the astral plane. But it was several years before I learned the comforting concepts of Yoga's anatomy of the many bodies (koshas). I lived through the experience without a philosophy or concept to understand it. It was a major revelation to know that I AM a consciousness that is independent of my physical body.

Over the next several months, I repeated the exercise of slowing down my breathing and heart until I could come and go from this realm, free of tension or anxiety. I learned how to relax in a way I would have never considered of interest or possible prior to this. I have found that this has produced a wonderful blessing - I am no longer afraid of death. I now know from this experience and many others that followed it, that I exist beyond the termination of my physical body. From that has arisen a tremendous serenity that remains present beneath the surface of all my activities.

XIV. Ayurvedic Yoga Natural Pranayama

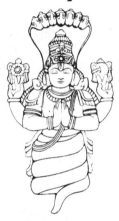

*"One who does not regulate the prana can have no attainment.
Control of the breath leads to control of prana."*
Swami Muktananda Paramahamsa

Ayurvedic Pranayama –
A word of caution

It is likely that you will experience that pranayamas and accessory techniques of mudra and bandhas vary from school to school and sometimes even from teacher to teacher in the same school.   One of the first considerations of learning pranayama is that every contemporary method presents it a unique manner. There is no standard method for achieving the goals of Pranayama practice. Indeed the goals themselves differ from school to school. Here I will focus on Pranayama in the context of Patanjali's guidelines with practical instruction following the instructions given by my teachers of Patanjali's Classical Yoga.

While other schools of yoga will differ from my methods presented, they are beneficial in helping the student progress toward the unique goals that the teacher seeks for the student. Among the most common differences with students learning pranayama in other methods will be that they were taught to breathe with the breath reversed that is filling the abdomen on the inhalation and lifting the breath upwards like filling a glass and exhaling in reverse of this. When seeing the disagreements that arise even from the basics of how to breathe, it is normal that confusion will arise. Students are cautioned to remember that learning pranayama in depth can only arise from being committed to only one school or better yet only one teacher. An ideal teacher is approved by their teacher and given guidelines for whom to teach and what practices they may present. Serious yoga students will understand this having integrity, reinforcing the vow (yama) of truthfulness (satya). For others who do not progress systematically due to lack of a teacher's guidance, they will have detriments instead of benefits. One could pretend to comprehend pranayama from a book or word of mouth of other students. This student will miss out on the wonderful blessings of pranayama as a crucial aspect of Yoga as a Path to Spirit. So seek a teacher, teachings and community who can support you in fulfilling your aspirations.

General Breathing Guidelines

Prior to formal training in Pranayama, students are taught how to breathe deeply consciously so that they can develop their sensitivities to feeling where the breath is most prominent. With few exceptions, most Yoga pranayamas are done only through the nostrils. The nasal passages are filled with subtle nerves that not only detect minor changes in temperature but also serve to heighten sensitivity, thus refining the balance of Vata. They also contain hair follicles designed to purify the air and lessen the tendency for colds and allergies to take hold.

Respiration changes as we age. Many people breathe with only one third of their respiratory capacity on a regular basis. Some of this change is due to poor posture that can produce atrophy in the spinal, abdominal and thoracic musculature. This in turn will make the ribcage less flexible, which in turn restricts breathing even more. Shallow breathing is a major contributing factor of diminished circulation, lack of energy, loss of memory, disorientation and confusion. It is a major factor in all disease and degenerative processes. Hence the restoration of full functioning can reverse or at the least lessen degeneration and disease symptomotology. The brain requires three times the amount of oxygen as other cells in the body. Inadequate oxygen can restrict the functioning of any of the vital organs. It is also symptomatic in feelings of anxiety (increased Vata) or depression (increased Kapha).

All of this can be turned around. By waking up your breathing, you will naturally heighten all physiological and psychological functions. Revolution and evolution are only a few inspired breaths away. Our mind trains our senses to restrict our attention to what it judges to be familiar, comfortable, and thus important. There is so much more taking place within the realm of the senses, let alone beyond them, that training can dramatically change your perception and interpretation of the events in your life. Yoga goes outside the norm. It is unnatural, mysterious and misunderstood; largely this is because we do not understand ourselves. Always remember that the process of Yoga and its goal of increasing self-knowledge are the same.

Begin breath training by watching the internal responses to breathe as you inhale. Feel free to exaggerate the feeling of expansion that is the hallmark of inspiration. The initial motion inward is sometimes accompanied with a slight flaring of the nostrils. This is fine to encourage in the beginning of your training. Along with this, one will more likely experience the qualities of the mucous lining of the nostrils; their degree of openness and how much whether or not moisture is present. This is the natural benefit of pranayama as it increases sensory nerve activity and heightens your ability to listen to your body's messages. It is a natural form of biofeedback. Provided your nostrils are clear, continue to pull your breath in as if smelling the aroma of a rose. If they are not clear, then clear them with tissue or practice warm water snuffing. This will create a more thorough and longer lasting opening.

Pull the air up from your nostrils until you can feel your sinus cavities. They are located above and behind your eyes. To facilitate this consciously, allow your upper body to relax. Tension of your face, neck, and shoulders diminishes respiratory awareness and you will also find the reverse to be true with practice. By increasing respiratory sensitivity, your upper body's muscular tensions will lessen. Encourage the inhaled air to move throughout the chambers of your cranial cavity. This may bring about sensitivities to areas you didn't believe air could possibly enter. It is highly recommended that you consult an anatomy atlas and become acquainted with the intricacy of the hollow spaces within your respiratory tract.[104] As you continue, you might feel some of the cool air enter the back portions of your mouth. Your ears may pop as pressure equalizes between the aural cavity and the oral cavity.

As the incoming air passes your oral cavity, it enters the trachea or windpipe on its way to your chest. In this region, there will sometimes be a sound arising from the throat as air passes over the voice box, the larynx and glottis just above the division of your bronchiole tubes. At this point, the windpipe separates from the esophagus, the smaller pathway for food located just behind your windpipe. If you have brought sufficient attention to this initial phase of emphasis on inspiration, you will experience tension continually leaving your upper body. This will produce the sensation of lightness indicative of balance in Apana Prana. However, if you are under chronic stress, your body may seem to be increasing in tension. As a result you might find that your shoulders are trying to kiss their cousins your ears. Additional tension may be experienced in your neck and head. Practice slow deep breathing until you can minimize the unwanted tensions outside of the respiratory channels.

Chronic stress is accompanied by inefficient use of the secondary muscles of respiration. These outer muscles of the shoulders, neck and chest become contracted with each and every breath taken. With this respiratory pattern, one cannot help feeling fatigued at the end of a normal day let alone a day that has unpredictable challenges. And what day doesn't?

The trachea divides into two downward and outward branches called bronchioles that lead to each lung. Your lungs fill up in all directions simultaneously though you might experience it in a number of possible sequences – from top to bottom, front to back, or center to periphery. The inhalation is caused by the downward motion of the diaphragm. This enormous muscle divides the upper third of your torso from the lower two thirds. Above the diaphragm are your lungs and heart, which receive the initial impressions of inspiration. The heart is attached to the diaphragm via the cardiac sac, which encloses it. It is not uncommon to feel your heart beating during the inhalation, as the heart is pulled downward and elongated. During the diaphragm's downward motion, it pushes upon the stomach, liver, adrenal glands, and kidneys, all of which lie immediately below it. As the diaphragm is attached to the internal wall of the ribcage, it pushes the ribs apart simultaneously lowering these upper abdominal organs toward the softer portions of the middle abdominal cavity. At the end of your full inhalation, you will feel your abdomen expanding and descending. A strong inhalation is a sign of healthy Adya Prana.

Inhalation Motions

For those untrained in harmonizing the diaphragm with their breath, the reverse is true. They experience the inhalation rising up from the abdomen then filling the chest. Most Yoga schools (except Krishnamacharya's lineage) teach breathing in this manner as it generates more of a relaxation response to focus motion into the abdominal cavity first. However, I find this method of breathing from the bottom up on the inhalation to be an inefficient movement, as it creates tension in the intercostal respiratory muscles located between the ribs. In assessing some of my clients with this breathing pattern I have found them to have chronic Vata imbalances such as back pain, menstrual cramps, and chronic fatigue.

In all my instruction in the Krishnamacharya lineage through his son Desikachar and the Russian "Mother of Yoga" Indra Devi, I learned to harmonize breath with motion. By changing to this method of feeling the respiratory wave, I have seen many of these clients improve their comfort and lessen or completely eliminate the symptoms they were having. Efficient respiration comes from maximizing the use of the internal muscles of the diaphragm and the two layers of intercostals muscles. For people with this breathing pattern, learning Yogic Breathing will take longer and require more attention to changing what was a reflex into a new habit.

Exhalation Motions

The exhalation is the reverse of the inhalation. Its motion is an ascending vertical flow of breath. It begins with a mild contraction in the lower abdominal muscles to propel carbon dioxide and waste gases up and out. The more forceful the exhalation the more forceful the abdominal contraction. During the mid range of exhalation, the lower rib cage narrows to assist with the ascent of the diaphragm. The exhalation comes steadily as a result of healthy Udana Prana.

For the Yogi the exhalation is the most emphasized aspect of breathing for through it we can generate the "Relaxation Response" as coined by Herbert Benson, MD and maintain serenity. The two major muscles controlling this motion are the diaphragm and the central or rectus abdominis. When done with deliberate conscious awareness, the exhalation can tone these muscles and cause a profound change in physiology. This change in turn changes our psychology. "The abdominal contraction has an effect on the parasympathetic nervous system. The vagus nerve (tenth cranial nerve) regulates much of the parasympathetic activity in the body. The vagus nerve attaches to the heart and is stimulated by the pressure initiated by the abdominal muscles pushing on the diaphragm and the heart during exhalation. This stimulation activates the parasympathetic nervous system to lower the heart rate, producing a calming effect." [105]

Intercostal Breathing

An exercise to assist in feeling the difference in the mid range is to place your palms curved around the ribcage as is shown above. Without any effort on the part of your arms, feel the changing shape of your ribs as you breathe fully. Notice how the inhalation increased the width of your ribcage and the exhalation narrows your circumference. The desired effect is an evenness of breath in three uppermost cavities of the body – abdominal, thoracic and cranial. For most people learning to allow the breath to become natural initially feels unnatural, perhaps even forced.

With consistent practice, you can recover the childlike natural motion of complete breathing that coordinates all the respiratory structures and musculature.

For a more advanced application of this technique see Pranayamas for Kapha.

The effect of full Yogic breathing upon the spine reveals the body's natural inclination to accompany movements with harmonized breathing. The motions of the ribcage during inhalation widen the chest, encouraging the arms to abduct and externally rotate from the shoulder girdle. As the diaphragm descends during inhalation, its lower tendons that are attached to the anterior bodies of the thoracic eleven and twelve vertebrae through the third lumbar vertebrae. The diaphragm exerts a pull that draws the lower spinal column forward. The psoas crosses over this lowest attachment of the diaphragm and will become contracted with it during inhalation. Together the two muscles contracting will create a mild backbend in the lower thoracic and upper lumbar region during full inhalation.

Anatomy books occasionally vary in their depiction of the diaphragm and psoas interface as they are drawn from cadavers and depict the fact that we are all unique. Just as we are different on the outside so are we different on the inside. I have seen drawings showing the overlap as little as two vertebrae to as much as five. The contraction of the psoas is accompanied by an external rotation of the femur from the hip socket. Thus, when the pelvis and legs are unrestrained during deep inhalation the entire torso can be experienced to be in a turned out, opening up, expansive, vulnerable posture. Along with this action, the superior pelvis will subtly rock forward (accentuating the backward bending tendency) as the lower front pelvis at the pubic region moves posteriorly. With a full inspiration, the rectus abdominis and other accessory respiratory muscles like the lateral abdominis oblique relax, allowing the abdominal organs to gently roll forward and downward. All these motions are experienced in an open body that allows respiration to be unhindered by external skeletal muscle tensions.

During the exhalation phase of breathing, there is a reversal of this tendency. The first motions include an ascending of the diaphragm that pulls the lumbar and lower thoracic regions posteriorly thus moving the torso into a mild forward bend. The thighs and pelvis rock into hip flexion and internal hip rotation with lumbar extension. In general, this creates a motion of the Child pose (Darnikasana). Emptying of the lungs collapses the chest. The shoulders move into internal rotation and the head moves into cervical flexion, forward and downward.

Summary of the Ayurvedic Yoga Breath

The inhalation using the Yogic Breath can be subdivided into three phases. During the initial motions, the breath enters the nostrils and descends via the trachea into the lungs, which will lift the chest and widen the upper rib cage. This phase stimulates Kapha seated in the chest region. The second phase consists of an intercostal motion as the middle and lower costal cartilage open to create a widening of the upper abdominal cavity. This phase stimulates Pitta whose home is the abdominal cavity. The third phase is a wavelike motion that descends from the downward moving diaphragm into the middle and lower abdominal cavity. This phase of the full breath stimulates Vata whose home is the true pelvic cavity.

This wave motion is hidden beneath the other two movements and at this phase of the complete breath, it stands out like the final waves of the ocean as they reach the shore. The analogy to the ocean's waves is fairly accurate as they also begin with a small yet powerful force, gathering momentum, and then in their middle phase, grow in amplitude and volume prior to peaking. Following the peak height, the waves are continuous ripples moving the smallest of particles and pushing them to new positions either back to the ocean (an Udana force) or removing them to distant regions of the shoreline away from the ocean (Apana force).

When all three phases of the Yogic Breath are done beautifully there is a tri-doshic effect. The mild stimulation of each dosha as it progresses through the cycle tends to restore homeostasis, which for the Yogi is the sattvic state. The need is to retain the evenness or sama vritti during the respiratory cycle so that the inhale and exhale are of the same force and duration. Once this is disturbed the doshas will also go into imbalance. When this is retained the doshas will create a deeper balance of the organism

Spontaneously Arising Pranayama and Bandhas

All Yogic techniques can be learned by a teacher who has experienced them spontaneously or from a teacher who learned precise ways to replicate what arose in their teacher. In the first method a spiritual awakening directs the practice from the inner teacher usually with clarification of the process coming from an outer teacher. This is a rare path. Some teachers who have been blessed with spontaneously arising Yoga include Amritanandamayi Ma (Ammachi - the hugging lady guru), Swami Muktananda of Ganeshpuri, Swami Kripalu, and Dhyan Yogi Madhusudandas. In most instances Yogic techniques are rather technical as they vary from one teacher to another who has not had the experience of the inner teacher directing the process. The differences amongst these paths are greater as the teachers focus on the outer teacher's methodology and not as much attention is given as to how to follow your inner teacher. In my writings, I am attempting to bridge the gap as I have received teachings from both inner and outer traditions.

While spontaneous asanas are not too common in contemporary yoga classes, they nonetheless happen. Similarly spontaneous pranayama will arise too. What I experience is that students who do their practice based on Patanjali's Classical Yoga guidelines adjust themselves so that their body's efforts in asana become sattvic and as a result, the breath flows more freely opening pranic pathways that others may not discover. As the body effort and energy align there will be inward drawing motions called bandhas. These "locks" open internal cavities and promote the retention of prana. In essence this locks the tri dosha qualities into their home cavities, not only balancing the doshas but also restoring the mind as prana to the sattvic guna.

Those students who are guided from within experience that their prana becomes awakened taking a new quality, which I call Shakti. Shakti is the energetic guidance of the inner teacher. When they take a selfless Ayurvedic Yoga inhalation a flow of Shakti will naturally arise from their humility and reverence. Each bodily cavity will react to the Shakti's motion creating a response that moves from pranayama to pratyahara (from outward to inward directed awareness). In the simple motion of inhalation, the head will move downward in such a manner as to create an upward tongue motion (Jiva bandha or Kechari mudra) accompanied by a neck lock (Jalandhara bandha). This is udana prana meeting and equalizing with adhya prana. The progression of the intercostal breathing pattern will bring about an expansion of the rib cage and with it an upward motion of the diaphragm (Uddiyana bandha). A very subtle lift of the pelvic floor (mula bandha) will arise at the end of the inhalation. This is samana prana meeting and equalizing with apana prana. A natural pause (kumbhaka) will follow as vyana prana expressing its nature before the exhalation. As the exhale proceeds to follow the reverse wave of the pranas, the bandhas will deepen from bottom to top resulting in a prolonged breath wave pause (kumbhaka) following the exhalation. Thus the naturally arising of bandhas as a manifestation of pratyahara (inward directed attention) will arise from the Ayurvedic Yoga Pranayama.

Unified the health benefits of Ayurveda in harmony with the naturally arising of spiritual desire creates a profoundly sattvic Yoga experience. The Shakti naturally brings one's attention to their inner teacher. Over time this process will deepen into a desire to share this sublime Shakti Shiva awareness with others who are seeking illumination. And often that sharing will arise without the student's effort.

Shakti loves to give Herself to good people. Good people will naturally have an increased prana, as that is the sign of the manifestation of their goodness. It is not merely the directing of life to the yogic lifestyle of ethical codes called yamas and niyamas. Practice is needed for those who do not experience Yoga naturally arising through all aspects of their life.

Pranayama Guidelines from the <u>Yoga Sutras</u>

The fourth limb of Patanjali's eight limbs of the tree of Yoga is Pranayama. Pranayama is defined in the first of four sutras (II, 49 – 53) citing that the experience of pranayama naturally follows the experience of asana.

> When this (asana mastery) is acquired
> then pranayama naturally follows
> with a cessation
> of the movements
> of inspiration and expiration. [106]

By taking this step we are entering the realm of the previously unknown. We are asked to suspend belief in the necessity of respiration as a requisite for life, as previously described in my experience of a spontaneous Yoga Nidra state. This stage of Yoga practice indeed calls for a leap in faith to allow our breath to suspend its constant motion and believe that we will still have life. Or it may come as a Spiritual awakening from a force higher than your personality's ego. Either way this limb calls for a letting go of the known and surrendering to the unknown. Here the Yogi enters the realm of the great mystery.

For others outside of these requisite conditions for pranayama, there is another way to gradually progress toward this fullness. Patanjali allows for the training of the breath as a means to allowing the requisite conditions for the higher form to gradually develop. The method is simple, yet sublime in its simplicity.

It is wonderful that we are so unique not only in outer form of physical body and posture but also inwardly. In my first seminar with Yoga master Desikachar in 1980 in San Francisco, he said, "God has established different rhythms for breath, pulse, brain unique to each person." The similarity that we all share is that we are unstable. And so by gradually gaining control over the vacillating nature of breath one can progressively visit the uncommon experience of stability. This can be done by regulating any of the breath's three principle qualities. It has the quality of moving external to the body during the exhalation (rechaka), moving internally during the inhalation (puraka), or it may be immobile during the natural pauses between movements (kumbhaka). According to Desikachar, the most important aspect of breath training is to increase the length of the exhalation.

The Yoga Sutras gives a practical progression for breath training to unveil the experience of pranayama.

II, 50
The vacillations of breath
are either external,
internal, or stationary,
they may be regulated
three ways:
by location, time, or number;
then they will become
prolonged and subtle. [107]

This practical sutra on pranayama training describes progression through following three steps. The first step in attaining pranayama according to Patanjali, is to direct your breathing to specific locations in the body and develop your capacity to restrain your attention to these specific regions. Thus in Yoga training, we begin with simple exercises to increase the expansion or contraction of the thoracic, abdominal, and pelvic cavity regions. Initially, this results in increased respiratory capacity, breath holding time, and sensitivity to the body's biofeedback mechanisms. With advanced training, the progression is to send the waves of the breath to subtler regions.

An example of progression would be to send the breath to the 4 cavities (cranial, thoracic, abdominal, and pelvic) then next to direct it within each cavity to a specific organ then to a region of that organ. For instance one could direct the breath to the abdominal cavity then to the posterior of that region, then to the kidneys and finally to the adrenal glands, located on top of the kidneys. With help from an anatomy atlas, one can begin to visualize smaller and more minute tissues until the prana of the breath can be directed to the level of cellular physiology.

The directing of the breath to specific areas of the physical body is a necessary prerequisite to effective healing. Through guided awareness by an adept teacher, the student can begin to sense the subtle physical motions of Prana within themselves. In this manner, blood flow can be increased to specific regions and, with practice, to internal organs. Studies of Yoga practitioners have demonstrated their capacity to alter the skin temperature in the hand as an indication of the ability to direct the flow of blood. Even novices can be taught to do this in a short period of time. Since many organ functions depend upon blood flow, increasing or diminishing circulation can have a profound effect upon health.

In the rarely published fifth chapter of the text <u>Hatha Yoga Pradipika</u>, the cultivation of awareness of Prana (Prana Dharana) is said to be a means to alleviating disease.

"Whenever any region is afflicted by disease one should contemplate upon the Vayu (Prana) situated in that region. . . . . Wherever there is affliction due to disease, filling that region (with Prana) one should hold it there." [108]

One meaning of the word prana is "that which is constantly present everywhere." Through this process of learning to direct the Prana into afflicted regions of the body, health improves. And with it the overall feeling of our innate interconnectedness increases. For it is this symmetry of experience that is Yoga. And with this phase of Yoga discipline the Pranayama discipline can be known as a means to that communion of Self. With that comes loss of the distinct sensations we call dis-ease. "True health is the unimpeded flow and containment of Prana within the body." [109]

The second method of training the breath is according to time or ratios. In the beginning the student is advised to concentrate primarily upon encouraging the flow of their breath to become full and smooth. This lessens the disruptions in the Prana as it moves into the five subdivisions. In general, certified Yoga teachers are advised to give only breath awareness or equal ratio (Sama Vritti "equal movement") breathing. This method is particularly beneficial in that it promotes concentration and steadiness of the body/mind during asana practice. It is free of the side effects that can arise from uneven breathing or training involving breath pauses. Variations to this standard are only ethically given individually by teachers authorized by their instructors to teach personal adaptations.

Uneven ratio (visama vritti "uneven motion") is given individually and then usually for a limited supervised period. This practice is highly beneficial for those persons with special needs. The effects of Yoga poses and pranayamas are classified as "fasting, contraction" (langhana) or "expanding" (brahmana). The most common change given from an even ratio is to extend the inhale. This promotes "expanding" of the lungs. By doing this, the digestion is stimulated as the lengthening of the inhalation stimulates Samana Prana. This in turn promotes more through elimination of waste products. There is also a general increase in digestive fire as Agni is increased by this prolonged inhalation.

This uneven pranayama is of particular benefit for those who desire to dive more deeply into meditation or who have irregular biological reflex patterns causing irregular menstrual cycles, constipation, and irregular sleep. This is especially beneficial for those with diagnosed problems in any region above the diaphragm. These practices should not be experimented with as they can disrupt the biological regulatory system of the hypothalamus. Some preliminary signals are obvious and should receive attention. When inhalation is increased too much there may be giddiness, hyperactivity, over reaction to sensory stimuli, weight gain, or suppression of grief and sadness.

In contrast with this, the lengthening of the exhalation is called "contracting" (langhana). It is easy for one to experience the principle of relaxation with a prolonged exhalation. The ribcage is narrow in width and depth during this phase of respiration. This variation in pranayama is utilized for those persons who are overworked, stressed or have excess tissue (increased Kapha). Caution is also needed in giving this practice due to detrimental side effects. With too much emphasis on exhalation there may be hyperventilation, dizziness from the increased expelling of toxins and, if habitually practiced, too much weight loss.

Taking these contrasting principles of langhana and brahmana as polarities of Yoga practice we can examine other polar opposites, which can be addressed by this practice. The following chart shows some examples of how to conceive of archetypal qualities that can also be used as guidelines for asana and mantra practices.

Brahmana - "to expand"	Langhana - "to fast"
Expansive	Constrictive
Lunar	Solar
Shakti	Shiva
Inhalation	Exhalation
Cooling	Heating - Agni
Nurturing & Tonifying	Detoxifying & Reducing
Kapha	Vata & Pitta
Forward bending	Backward bending

The third discipline applied to the breath is the number. This refers to the number of cycles or minutes that a particular method is performed. Gradually the amount of time spent is increased until the range of control over the respiratory function is extended to double your initial practice.

In this way, the breath regulation can be carried out for periods that will help restore biological and circadian rhythms to homeostasis. As Vata regulates all motions in the body/mind, this alteration of respiration will deepen the changes to all life rhythms. This is a particularly beneficial intervention for those undergoing changes in life – birth, menopause, mid-life crisis, moving to a new city, change in job or relationship. Regulating the number of the breaths can assist the individual's capacity to adapt to larger changes. Once more we see how manipulating the microcosm can assist in adapting to changes in the macrocosm.

This will usually allow sufficient time for the student to discover the difference between breathing exercise and pranayama. This distinction is learned by experience of the waves of Prana rather than through understanding.

When this training becomes stable for 5 minutes, you may begin the second phase of practice – extending the natural length of each breath. This follows with the second definition of pran-ayama in <u>Yoga Sutras</u> II, 51-52. Drawing out the breath deepens one's ability to concentrate and maintain a still posture. The breath becomes more subtle and the Pranic energy in the breath becomes more apparent.

Pranayama practice is a tremendous tool for expanded awareness and yet for many students, a taste of this expansion is enough. They may stop and not proceed further in the development of the potentials of Pranayama. For this heightened self awareness often points out areas of life that are stressful – where they experience a lack of empowerment or where they are fearful of change. The process of self-awareness that Pranayama affords can produce radical change in lives that are stuck due to an unmanageable lifestyle, lost motivation or inspiration. It seems peculiar and overly simplistic that by just working with your respiratory inspiration you can also increase your psychic and mental inspiration and live a more fulfilling life. It is due to this challenge that a serious Yogini receives the title of Hero (Vira). For being a committed Yogini reveals bravery to face the challenges of your own self. Taking the vows of regular Yoga sadhana brings courage and by its development more is given.

Asanas for Pranayama

While the majority of my pranayamas are done in seated postures; two, agnisar dhouti and Uddiyana bandha, are done from a standing posture with hands on bent knees. Although any comfortable posture with the pelvic sitz bones 6" higher than your knees is suitable for pranayama, I do have my preferences of poses. It is ideal to use the best-seated posture you can do that locks your legs and pelvis into a static posture. My other favorite postures, in order, equal pose (Samasana), auspicious pose (Swastikasana) or easy pose (Sukhasana). Samasana is with the left heel to the perineum for women and right foot in front of it, both feet flat on the ground, heels centered on the pelvis. Swastikasana is done with the right foot resting between the left calf and thigh. Sukhasana has the ankles crossed feet pointed ahead and placed directly below the knees so the lower legs are supported by the opposite ankles.

Once your legs are comfortably positioned, and then create an erect spine using strong back muscles to lift your chest and head to an elongated posture. Then begin with your arms fully extended, hands palm down in Chin mudra (consciousness gesture or seal) or palms upward in Jnana mudra (wisdom), lightly touching thumb and forefinger tips. Anjali mudra with palms at the heart or any other mudra you prefer can also be beneficial. These gestures will help produce the attitude of mind for expanding consciousness into the fourth kosha, subtler than the mind's normal states. When considered as seals they help the Yogini to retain/seal pranic flows that otherwise may escape the subtle nadis of the hands and feet. Overtime pranic nadis are built to generate and sustain higher states of consciousness until the highest (fourth) procedure of prana is attained where prana is felt permeating everywhere as the veil over the pure light of consciousness is lifted (YS II, 51-2).

Sequence for Learning Pranayamas

Although I have listed these pranayamas in the Ayurvedic sequence of Vata, Pitta, and then Kapha balancing; the sequence to learn them in is different. Optimal is to learn ujjaye first, nadi shodhana Kriya second, intercostal breathing third, agnisar dhouti fourth, Kapalabhati Kriya fifth, Sitali sixth, and Shambhavi Bhastrika last. In this way the abdominal and respiratory muscles can gradually be toned to the level required by the most demanding of the practices, Shambhavi Bhastrika.

Pranayama for Vata

In general, pranayama balances Vata and calms the mind. Eight types of pranayama are described in the classical 14th century text <u>Hatha Yoga Pradipika</u> (II, 44-70). The safest are cited here. As a reminder, before any pranayama practice, the purification technique of Water Snuffing (Jala Neti) described in chapter 6 is recommended to be done to open the sinus and upper respiratory passages clearing them of excess mucous.

Even Wave Victorious - Sama Vritti Ujjaye

Described in detail in my previous book, <u>Structural Yoga Therapy</u>, as the wave breath, this is the most natural discipline of the Prana to engage in continuously. Sama means even. Vritti means vacillation or wave. Ujjaye comes from two root words, uj meaning "upward" and jayi meaning "victorious." It is a wave motion of breath that raises consciousness and frees the mind from delusions and self-centeredness, allowing the Truth to be known and acted upon.

The principle characteristic of this pranayama is even inhale and exhale, even duration, even effort. Gradually natural pauses (Kumbhakas) are introduced.

Following the guidelines of Patanjali <u>Yoga Sutras</u> II, 50 the prana is to become "prolonged and subtle" by this even, sattvic effort. Ujjaye can also be translated to mean, "what clears the throat and masters the chest region." An important technique for Hatha Yoga, Ujjaye is a glottal breath in which the back of the throat is partially closed to narrow the passage of air entering the windpipe (trachea). Ujjaye is the basic pranayama technique from which all others derive.

Precautions

There are no contraindicated conditions for which to deny oneself this practice. Even actively deranged doshas will benefit from attempts at regulating prana through this foundational pranayama.

Common Problems

The most often is stressful breathing, efforting to perfect the posture, too tight a neck position and tensions of the upper body are common with rajasic practitioners.

Instructions

The optimal posture is seated meditation position with your back erect and head slightly bent down, bowing toward your heart. Your head is tilted not contracted downward enough to form Chin Lock (Jalandhara bandha), but enough to create the sensation of the trachea narrowing in the region of the glottis. The posture gives one the attitude of humility. I call the muscles creating this bowing pose, the humility muscles. They are rarely strong enough to sustain the position for a serious pranayama practice. The chest/heart is raised to allow your lungs the freedom to easily expand. Place your hands palm up on your knees with the tips of your forefinger and thumbs joined in Wisdom's Seal, Jnana Mudra, and your arms straight.

The technique is done by inhaling smoothly and evening through both nostrils. Then follows a brief pause. Exhalation should be done through both nostrils. The primary method is done with evenness of inhalation and exhalation (technically called sama vritti ujjaye pranayama). Its primary benefit is to balance all the aspects of Vata's five pranas and prepare the mind for withdrawing from the world (pratyahara) into concentration (dharana). Place your attention on the breath sound. Inhale and exhalation is through both nostrils. The inhale and exhale are maintained at an even, steady pace. A constriction will be created at the base of your throat that makes the sound more audible.

Begin by taking a deep breath and feel with your fingertips the soft juncture of skin above and between your collarbones (clavicles) sinking in. It is from this contraction that the "hamm" sound arises. With concentration, the sound can become even and sustained from the beginning to the end of each inhale. Over time this sound will also become articulated during the exhalation cycle as well. There is no pause with the breath, only a smooth, steady in-out flowing cycle. The main qualities of the breath are the vertical motions of the breath's wave and its subtle throat sound.

Benefits

By persistently following the <u>Yoga Sutra</u> guidelines this practice creates the state of pranayama and the experiences cited in II, 49-52. This practice overtime leads to an inward directed awareness that continuously perceives the currents of sensation that are the essence of prana. It is a breathing that allows consciousness to rise courageously above its usually restless mental nature and through that victory to experience the underlying transcendental Self. The mind then becomes calm, and the stillness, which is always there beneath your thoughts surface with clarity.

Variation for attaining higher consciousness

Cultivate devotion (Bhakti) seeking the Divine Presence as pure awareness. In this case that Presence is the awareness of breath. Feel with great sensitivity the sensations of the singular air from the outside becoming two as it enters the separate left (ida) and right (Pingala) channels. Notice just beyond the root of the nostrils the breath that was two becomes one. Then breathe out to experience the twoness again. Watch very carefully the turning points where one becomes two and two becomes one. This method comes from the Vijnana Bhairava Tantra sutras 24, 25, and 27. [110]

Purifying the Subtle Energy Channels - Nadi shodhana

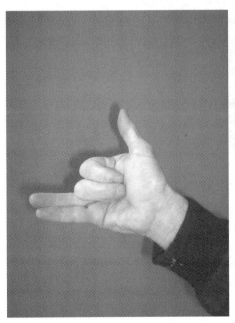 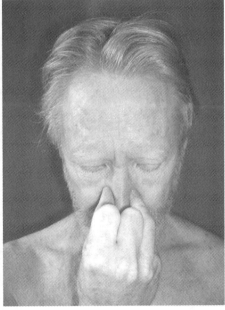

"The yogi who has thus overcome fatigue by practicing the asanas, should begin practice of purification of the subtle nerve, the nadis, manipulation of prana, pranayama and mudras to introvert the subtle energies in order to deepen meditation practice." [111]

The purification of the nadis occurs through all pranayama practices though the practice of alternate nostril breathing is especially renowned for this benefit. This is an example of how each Yoga system is unique. In writing a forward to his student's guidebook on the distinctions of Asana and Pranayama in his tradition, T.K.V. Desikachar notes "there are no standards for names or techniques of each asana and pranayama." [112] It is known in different Yoga systems as either nadi shodhana (purification of the subtle channels) or anuloma viloma (alternating the current). This technique consists of altering the side of inhalation and exhalation. Without breath retention (kumbhaka), this is called nadi shodhana. This is the safest way to begin practice. For those with regular pranayama practices, the addition of breath retention following each motion changes its nature and therefore, its name. In this variation, it is known as anuloma viloma.

It is described in <u>Hatha Yoga Pradipika</u> II, 7-13. This alternate nostril breathing is recommended prior to other pranayamas and before meditation practice.

"When all the nadis and chakras (which are full of impurities) are purified, then the yogi is able to retain prana." [113]

By alternately breathing through each nostril, the mind naturally begins to find the state of peace and one's attention goes inward.

Precautions

The main side affect to avoid is dizziness or lightheadedness. This may arise from going to rapidly or from trying to force open a closed nostril. Be sure you do water snuffing (see chapter 6) should the alternating nostrils feel restricted.

Instructions

This pranayama is performed by closing alternate nostrils. First the right palm is spread open and the index finger and middle fingers are turned down to rest at the base of the mount of Venus muscle formation beneath the thumb. The ring, little finger and the thumb remain extended. This hand position is called Doe Seal (Mrigee Mudra) although in some circles is called Vishnu Mudra. It is used to regulate the opening and closing of the nostrils. Then place the right thumb along side the middle ridge of the bone of the right nostril midway from the cheekbone to the top of the nose so that the tip of the ring finger can apply equal pressure on the left middle nasal bone.

The ideal placement will press a sensitive point half way from the bridge of the nose to the cheekbone along the edge of the lateral nasal bones. The thumb and ring finger tip should remain in contact with these points throughout the practice.

Do not remove your fingers from your nose. Then alternately vary the pressure from side to side to close the right then the left nostril using a subtle sideways wrist motion called radial then ulnar deviation. [114]

Begin with your hand in position with a mild pressure applied to both nasal points. Practice Ujjaye breathing for some time through both nostrils until you are comfortable with your hand in this position. Keep your spine straight and head centered, slightly bowed. Correct any tendency to turn your head toward your right. Bring your hand toward your head rather than the reverse. Then begin to alternate currents, inhaling through the left nostril, slowly yet fully. Change pressure to exhale through the right nostril. Then inhale through the right nostril. Change and exhale through the left. This ends one round, continue for 6-10 rounds, and then sit quietly allowing your mind to experience the spaciousness that arises from balancing the channels of respiration.

Practice Ujjaye breathing for some time through both nostrils until you are comfortable with your hand in this position. Keep your spine straight and head centered, slightly bowed. Correct any tendency to turn your head toward your right. Bring your hand toward your head rather than the reverse.

Then begin to alternate currents, inhaling through the left nostril, slowly yet fully. Change pressure to exhale through the right nostril. Then inhale through the right nostril. Change and exhale through the left. This ends one round, continue for 6-10 rounds, and then sit quietly allowing your mind to experience the spaciousness that arises from balancing the channels of respiration.

Variations

The next level of practice is directing your Prana to specific physical regions such as feeling the breath in the cranial, then thoracic then abdominal then pelvic cavities. Then create an awareness that extends to each of these cavities. Practice gradually extending the duration of your breath without stress or strain. The purpose is to slow down your breath with only minor changes in lowering heart rate or blood pressure.

A second variation can be done with the addition of breath pauses (kumbhaka) following each motion changes its benefits and its name is anuloma viloma. This name means *"alternating currents."* This is especially potent in uncovering the subtle, all pervasive nature of prana known as Adya (or the primary) Prana. The pause should at first be only half the duration of the motions. That is inhaling and exhaling for a count of 8 can be alternated with pauses of 4. The best form of kumbhaka is the naturally arising form. In this way the True Self reveals itself in a sattvic manner without even the slightest rajasic tendency of effort.

Benefits

"When all the nadis and chakras (which are full of impurities) are purified,
then the yogi is able to retain prana." [115]

The ability to retain prana is a great achievement. Many people are basically like leaky buckets with their life force on any or all dimensions (koshas). By practicing this technique the practice moves from Hatha Yoga to its subtle body benefits that is the hallmark of Tantrik Yoga. Classical Yoga of the medieval period did not distinguish Hatha from Tantra Yoga or Raja Yoga. They were all considered as one yoga according to the Hatha Yoga Pradipika, IV, 103.

Pranayama for Pitta

Cleansing the Fire - Agnisar Dhouti

This practice is given previously as one of the Six Purification Methods (see chapter 6). Review the notes there in your practice and then consider these additional comments to deepen your practice from a Kriya to a Pranayama.

Agni creates a physical purification by increasing the movement of air in the fire region of the middle abdomen. We all know that our body temperature is naturally 98.6° F. This is remarkable that our body maintains such a high internal heat in spite of what the weather is like outside. Agni is responsible for that heat maintenance. Water coming into our body at the mouth is cooler than that exiting the urinary canal via the urethra. An ideal sign of balance of this Agni as a sub form of Pitta is that the belly will feel to be the warmest place on the skin.

Precautions

This practice, like other abdominal exercises such as Kapalabhati, nauli, and Uddiyana Bandha, is not recommended for menstruating women or those who are pregnant; as well as persons suffering from respiratory or cardiovascular disease, ulcer, hiatal hernia, or abdominal disorders. It is best done one hour prior to a meal or at least two hours following a meal. If recovery from each repetition takes more than three breaths, you are straining your internal organs and going beyond your current capacity. Remember to be gentle with abdominal exercises.

Common Errors

The pulling and releasing should be applied directly back and forth, unlike Uddiyana Bandha, in which the pull is exerted back and upward, resulting in a hollow upper abdominal cavity. It is important to keep your head down both to maintain a neck lock, and to watch the motions to your central abdomen. It is imperative that the inward pull of the belly occurs only during exhalations; otherwise headaches and dizziness may result. Keep your upper body stationary without lifting your shoulders, tensing your neck, or dropping your chest. For the benefits to accrue the practice should be centered on the central abdomen.

Instructions

Once you have learned to isolate your torso so that it does not move during the practice, you can begin to expand the benefits to the subtle body. The best way to learn this practice is from a standing position. Prepare yourself by baring your abdomen so you can observe its movements throughout the practice. From this posture spread your feet slightly wider than hip distance and bend your knees, while keeping the back in neutral spinal alignment with a lumbar curve. Place your hands above your knees with straight arms. This will enable you to hold your torso and shoulders still. Tilt your head downward and watch your abdomen throughout the exercise. It is important that you keep your eyes open and observe the motions so that you can focalize them to the navel region. If you cannot see the belly due to large chest then you may place a mirror on the floor in front of and between your feet and gaze there.

Inhale, relax your abdomen letting its contour fall forward with gravity, and then exhale pulling the central abdominal region straight backward (NOT upwards as in Uddiyana Bandha). Repeat this preliminary practice of abdominal breathing six times, then inhale deeply and while exhaling lower your head until your chin is close to your chest forming the neck lock (Jalandhara Bandha). While holding the breath out, gently pull the belly back and relax it repeatedly in a comfortable steady pace until you run out of air.

Then release the neck lock and slowly inhale returning to normal abdominal breathing while continuing to observe the belly. Your holding time will be about 20-30 seconds so as to not strain any of the respiratory muscles or heart.

Repeat the procedure after taking a minimum of three slow breaths to create an effect of gently massaging your abdominal organs. For the next repetitions count the number of contractions you can sustain and strive for a number and pace that is stable. I am assuming that you are having no side affects and have thoroughly read the cautions. The neck lock action will assist at prolonging the breath pause without strain.

To enhance the benefits of the practice visualize that deep within your abdomen is a fireplace and the motions of your abdomen are fanning the fire to increase your digestive heat. Allow any excess heat to escape up the chimney through your upper body. When balanced the warmest area of your body as felt by your palm will be your belly.

When you need to breathe be sure to allow your abdomen to move naturally in harmony with your breathing.

Benefits
Regular practice increases the strength of your abdominals, and improves stamina by the increase in your breath holding time. This practice decreases Kledaka Kapha. It increases Pachaka Pitta and Agni and therefore improves digestion. For students who are overweight consistent practice can assist a more balanced diet in regaining your constitutional body size. Dhouti is for most any kind of digestive tract trouble. There are a few conditions that precautions are needed for its use but the main consideration is simply doing the practice correctly. This is the only Dhouti that I recommend for everyone to learn. Learning this is a prerequisite for learning Uddiyana bandha, the stomach lock.

It also helps you get over your attachment to your body. I've used it for that as well. All of these Vata balancing techniques are also very useful for people with addictions. Drug addictions, alcohol addictions, and behavioral addictions are lightened by this type of Kriyas. Dhouti, if used for addictions, has to be supervised. Remember, there are multi-dimensions to this body. All addictions have their root in the mind but they flower in the body. So, every single illness, every single illness; there is no illness which is an exception to this rule. There is no mental or physical ailment that does not have its root in Vata. That's the core issue. There are three related pranayamas – Agnisar Dhouti, Kapalabhati, and Bhastrika. The optimal learning procedure is to learn Agnisar Dhouti Kriya first followed by the others in the sequence above. Learning them in this order minimizes the incidence of potential side effects.

Cooling Breath - Sitali
This practice is a way to curb excess Pitta. It is described in Classical Hatha Yoga texts, Hatha Yoga Pradipika II, 57-58 and Gheranda Samhita V, 73-74.

Precautions
Practice this pranayama no more than one minute, except under the guidance of a Yoga Therapist (especially if you seek to use it for its Pitta reducing properties).

Instructions
Exhale then protrude your tongue just beyond your lips. Fold the edges of your tongue up forming a trough shape. The ability to curl the tongue is passed on as a genetic factor, so not everyone can do it. If you cannot curl your tongue, instead make a circle with your lips as you would to suck liquid through a straw. Then narrow the passage by pressing your lips around your folded tongue. Inhale and direct the cooling effect of your inhalation to the posterior wall of your oral cavity. Feel it reaching down your trachea extending into your chest region. Then, close your mouth and exhale through both nostrils.

It is not necessary to fold the tongue for the technique to work adequately to cool you. The key is the ability to draw the coolness from the air and take it deeply down through your chest energetically reaching the fire chakra of your belly. The practice is best done for short periods of time, about 1-2 minutes are sufficient.

Benefits
In the summer, a longer practice of up to two minutes is recommended as it can dramatically reduce your body's excessive heat buildup. This pranayama reduces excess Pitta dosha. The Hatha Yoga Pradipika II, 58 claims that it "can cure swelling of the stomach, spleen, fever, excess bile, hunger and counteracts poisons."

Variation
A variation that was given by my teacher from his individual sessions with

Krishnamacharya consists of slowly raising your head as you inhale. At the top of the inhalation, a cool column of air will be felt extending deeply into your abdomen. Then pause while lowering your chin towards your chest, stopping just shy of applying a Neck Lock (Jalandhara Bandha). With your head downward, exhale slowly through both nostrils. Consciously release any sense of excess heat from your body. Pause before continuing with the next inhalation. This variation is an ideal way to learn to apply Neck Lock gradually yet fully in harmony with the other bandhas. This practice can be extended for 2-5 minutes. It is wonderfully soothing during the intensity of the heat of summer. This reduces Pitta dosha as it restores balance to the Vata dosha.

Bellows - Bhastrika

After learning to do Agnisar Dhouti and Kapalabhati (described under Pranayamas for Kapha) so that you can experience the distinct differences in their benefits, then Bellows pranayama can be safely learned. Bhastrika Pranayama (described in the <u>Hathayoga Pradipika</u> II, 59-67 and the <u>Gheranda Samhita</u> V, 75-77) is characterized by a quick expulsion of breath producing a sound like a fireplace bellow. The practice is a continuation of training that was begun with Kapalabhati Kriya in chapter 6.

Precautions

See previous notes, as the precautions are the same as for Agnisar Dhouti and Shambhavi Bhastrika. Students who have not properly prepared with the preliminary practices are more likely to have adverse side effects of headaches or inflammation of excessive Pitta symptoms. It is imperative that the inward pull of the belly occurs only during exhalations; otherwise headaches and dizziness may result. Keep your upper body stationary without lifting your shoulders, tensing your neck, or dropping your chest. For the benefits to accrue the practice should be centered on the abdomen.

The practice is quite powerful and needs to be done for a brief period as described. Prolonged practice can awaken more energy than one is capable of using. While its use can be done for those on long retreat or living in a spiritual community, it is not advised to do regular practice with a householder 9-5 work schedule.

Common Errors

Flexing the spine and shoulders during the motions are signs of inadequate preparation. The experienced yoga student will be able to isolate motions to specific regions of the body. In this case we seek a statue like posture with the motions isolated to the central abdominal cavity.

Instructions

For the first level of practice begin as in Kapalabhati, exhaling with even paced, forcible contractions of the central abdomen. Allow the inhalation to occur without effort. The amount of force on the exhalation is moderate yet insufficient to flare the nostrils or create tensions in the neck or facial muscles. Your posture will remain stable and relatively motionless once your practice is proficient.

First carry out a few rounds of even-paced Kapalabhati. Practice to your capacity, but not more than 60 seconds. Then after the last expulsion take a deep inhalation followed by the pause and apply first the Root Lock then the Neck Lock. Hold the pause as long as is comfortable, then let the exhalation release slowly and gently without strain. This is one round of Bhastrika. Practice no more than three rounds without a qualified supervisor to guide you.

Benefits

Pitta practices are invariably purifying and the bringing up of these impurities may elicit physical or emotional symptoms. Bhastrika Pranayama increases Agni and Pachaka Pitta.

The raising of anxiety, depression and fear are among the most common side effects of an effective pranayama practice. Through persistence, faith in a higher power, and good guidance these are overcome.

Variation

Bellows of the Goddess – Shambhavi Bhastrika

This technique came from my spiritual teacher who approved my sharing of this unique and profound practice. Shambhavi means the Goddess; She is both the consort that accompanies Her Lord as Shiva and his left side when they are one

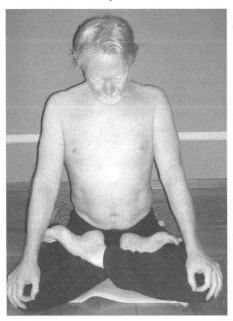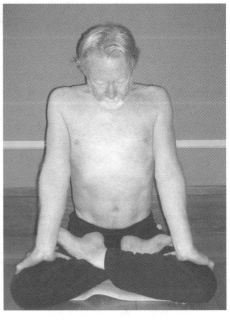

body. When they are harmonious, She is the Goddess governing all movement. In this form she is the awakened prana called Shakti. Her nature is the luminous light that accompanies Siva's stillness. His nature is pure consciousness from which springs Her motion of thought and its apparent worldliness. It may seem a paradox that stillness is characterized by having tremendous energy but it is the natural order of the universe that there be a balance of opposites.

There are many variations that are to be learned from a qualified pranayama teacher as this practice can profoundly deepen meditation as a result of the enhanced purification of the nadis that this more profound practice elicits. Once developed this practice can catapult the student into a deep meditation without the normal need to direct your thoughts to a specific technique. This variation increases the efficiency of Bhastrika to create a profoundly still meditative state (Siva consciousness).

Precautions
The same considerations apply as to Bhastrika, agnisar dhouti, and kapalabhati.

Instructions
The ideal posture for Shambhavi Bhastrika is Lotus (Padmasana). Since this practice can bring out the deeper impurities of both the physical and psychic body, the Lotus posture can help one to rise above any uncomfortable sensations that are bound to arise from its continued practice.

Like all pranayama practices, they need to be given by a teacher who was trained to spread it by their teacher. In this case, to be authorized to teach it Swami Muktananda's staff had to teach it while seated in full lotus (Padmasana), with the left foot on top. For all others who do not wish to be certified by Mukunda to teach this, it can be practiced from any comfortable posture with the pelvic sitz bones 6" higher than your knees. It is ideal to use the best seated posture you can do, one that locks your legs and pelvis into a stable support for a static posture. My other favorite postures, in order, equal pose (Samasana), auspicious pose (Swastikasana) or easy pose (Sukhasana). Samasana is with the left heel to the perineum for women and right foot in front of it, both feet flat on the ground, heels centered on the pelvis. Swastikasana is done with the right foot resting between the left calf and thigh. Sukhasana has the ankles crossed feet pointing ahead so they are directly below the shins so the lower legs are supported by the opposite ankles.

Exaggerate your erect spine using strong back muscles and begin with arms fully extended hands palm down in chin mudra, lightly touching thumb and forefinger tips. The practice is similar to kapalabhati Kriya, except that the pace is faster and the intention is to bring Pitta home to the central belly. This will result in a warmer central abdomen more than any other part of the body.

Begin with an exaggerated abdominal breathing so that every exhalation is accompanied by a central abdominal contraction. The inhalations are with relaxation of the abdomen. After 3 or more abdominal breaths do short, sharp exhalations while maintaining steadiness of pacing at a faster rate than normal Bhastrika. After 30 seconds of sustained breathing, exhale fully. As you inhale form a strong reverse elbow lock by turning your palms flat at the end of your thighs with fingers pointing toward your body. If your body proportions do not permit this then the palms can be placed fingers reversed on the floor in front of your shins. Then pull your shoulders back and downward while extending the spinal column so that your entire ribcage will be fully lifted. Next exhale fully as you apply the triple bandhas from root to abdominal to neck lock. Gradually equalize the effort amongst them.

Concentrate your inner awareness on your heart opening and seeing the Goddess within. Retain the breath as long as it feels natural. When the impulse to breathe comes, release the bandhas and locked arms slowly as you inhale gently allowing your lungs to fill. Sit quietly allowing the breath to return in its own rhythm. It will tend to be quite slow as your prana and its thoughts will also move very slowly. This can be repeated up to three times prior to meditation practice.

Benefits
It balances all the doshas when done well and increases udana prana leading to a deep state of Siva and Shambhavi consciousness. A natural state of meditation arises when both the effort and the surrender to the benefits is harmonious with sattva guna being predominant.

Pranayama for Kapha

Intercostal Breathing
This was described earlier as the middle component (that is the range of the space between the diaphragm and the base of the ribcage) of the complete breath. With practice at isolating this motion, it can become a more powerful tool for elevating your energy levels. To expand your midrange place your hands curved around the shape of your lower ribcage, as shown below. Exhale and press the fingertips together so that they meet adjacent to your solar plexus. Inhale and expand the region beneath your hands. As you exhale begin to press mildly with your hands to emphasize the narrowing of your ribcage. Adjust the width of your hands to let the middle fingertips lightly touch at the end of your exhale. Inhale expanding outward with your ribs, which will strengthen your external intercostal muscles. Exhale using the strength of your arms to narrow the ribs while contracting the internal intercostal muscles.

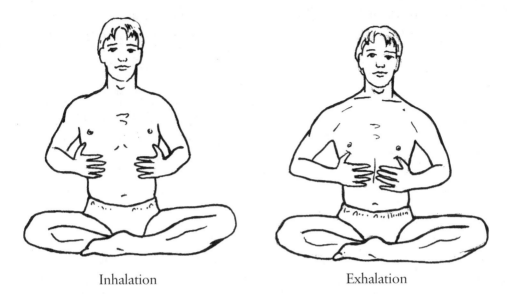

Inhalation   Exhalation

To make the exercise more effective resist the motions of your intercostal muscles with your hands as you inhale. Let it be a moderate tug of war in which your intercostals will win. This will give them resistance to work with and will increase your inspiratory strength. Then reverse the procedure so that the intercostals will resist the pressing inward of the ribs as you exhale pushing with your hands. Let your hands win.

Continue and notice how much expansion you can get with each inhalation. Ideal is to have 2-3 inches of expansion at the lower sternal region. You can get a cloth tape measure to determine the difference between the circumference of the inhalation and that of exhalation. A standard I have for yoga teachers is to have 3 inches of increased circumference and for Yoga Therapists, 4 inches. In this manner the opening of the Kapha region at the heart can be shown to have a physical component.

The Flying Stomach Lock – Uddiyana Bandha

Uddiyana Bandha, which literally translated means the "flying up lock", is more commonly called the stomach lock. It is given this name as it increases the activity of Udana Prana whose natural motion is an upward motion through the upper torso and head. This is the third bandha to be learned; first neck lock then root lock. It consists of a strong abdominal contraction that will create a vacuum in the upper abdomen following complete exhalation. There are several phases of its development (see notes on Nauli Shatkarma).

Precautions

The same precautions apply as to agnisar dhouti, kapalabhati, and Shambhavi Mudra. Women are cautioned not to do this practice if menstruating or pregnant.

It is unsafe for others with heart conditions, hiatal hernia, ulcers, or respiratory conditions. It is safe to do this exercise in the early morning or in the hour preceding a meal.

Common Errors

The most common problems are doing the practice with the breath reversed that is abdomen going out on exhalation, and holding the breath (kumbhaka) after inhalation then doing the bandha. While in other schools this may be the way it is taught, this differs from my method. Students are cautioned to remember that pranayamas and the accessory techniques of mudra and bandhas vary from school to school and sometimes even from teacher to teacher in the same school.

Instructions

In the first phase the student will have been practicing Agnisar Dhouti for some time and has developed the capacity to hold the in breath while rhythmically contracting the abdominals thirty times. When this is done comfortably without stress upon the heart as indicated by palpitations or without a sudden rush of incoming air then the stomach lock can be applied. Following the execution of half a normal round of Agnisar Dhouti, the abdomen is pulled backward in an exaggerated fashion and held in this position. This will create a hollow of the middle and upper abdominal cavity. This is to be repeated three times with natural breathing in between rounds.

In the second phase, the Neck Lock (Jalandhara Bandha) is applied first then the abdominal contraction is applied with a strong back then upward pull. With this phase, there should be a lifting of the diaphragm and an expansion of the ribcage to create the hollow of the upper abdominal region. The "flying up" of the diaphragm having been achieved for 10-15 seconds, the muscles are slowly released followed by an inhalation. This is to be repeated three times while allowing for as many breaths to be taken as necessary for recovery to take place in between rounds. Once the student has built up their stamina, the breath holding time can be increased to up to thirty seconds. This is provided that the inhalation following the release is smooth and not strained.

Benefits

The Stomach Lock produces a profound change to the abdominal contents. The air in the hollow digestive organs of the large and small intestines and to a lesser extent the stomach is pushed out. The earliest physiological studies of Yoga were undertaken in 1926 at the Kaivalyadhama Yoga Research Institute reporting on the internal pressure changes as a result of Uddiyana Bandha. Their findings reveal a vacuum created in the lower cavities of the large intestine created by the strong upward pull of the diaphragm. The increased diameter of the ribcage allowed the upper abdominal organs to be displaced into the thoracic cavity. It is believed that the muscular walls of the intestines were collapsed as x-rays done following barium enema showed a radical change in the normal shape of these organs.

Its therapeutic application includes indigestion, excess wind, constipation, irregular appetite and incontinence. Once developed it can also be of benefit to respiratory ailments as it can increase the power of both exhalation and inhalation. It is regarded as an important element in the treatment of asthma.

Regular practice reduces excess weight and balances Kledaka and Tarpaka Kapha. It also stimulates the digestive fire, Jatharagni, which may result in improved metabolism and improved elimination. Regular practice can create an aura of lightness and bring clarity to your mind. It is also renowned for relieving respiratory conditions, colds, eyestrain, allergies and other conditions that may be influenced by changes of the seasons or the quality of mucous in the linings of the nasal and sinus passages.

Shining the Skull - Kapalabhati Kriya

This practice is one of the Shatkarmas as introduced in chapter six. Here I will introduce more advance concepts from the Shatkarma Kriya technique given previously. The term kapalabhati literally translates to the "head shining" practice. As a purification practice it acts like water snuffing clearing your head and respiratory passages by expelling excess mucous. It is a good idea to keep a tissue handy in the event that you are successful.

As a pranayama it literally manifests the meaning of the Sanskrit word. Thus it generates an internalization of prana that reveals the light body of the head.

Precautions

See previous notes, as the precautions are the same as for Agnisar Dhouti and Shambhavi Bhastrika. For the benefits to accrue the practice should be centered on the abdomen with the posture remaining statue like. For adequate preparation the student needs to be practicing regularly 6 rounds of 30 agnisar dhouti practice with no side affects.

Common Errors

Similar to agnisar dhouti, it is common to not be able to isolate the motions of the abdomen with the rapid breathing, resulting in flexing the spine and shoulders during the motions.

Instructions

It is ideal to first do water snuffing then kapalabhati. The breath is done only in a stable seated position. It consists of short, sharp abdominal contractions during each exhalation done rhythmically at the pace of one per second. The air is inhaled without effort to return the abdomen to its normal position. Begin with a hand placed palm up upon your knee in Jnana Mudra (Wisdom Seal). Place your other palm on the middle of your abdomen. Begin with a natural breathing pace and make sure that your abdomen contracts away drawing your hand toward the back with each exhalation. After a minute begin to contract your navel region more markedly on the exhalation while allowing your muscles to relax to normal position for the inhalation. The focus is upon a strong exhalation while allowing the inhalations to come naturally between them.

After the coordinated motion is maintained then you can begin to do the practice pacing each exhalation gradually faster until the rate of 1 breath per second is established. Condition yourself to be able to reach 30 seconds of sustained practice. If the rhythm cannot be maintained then a shorter quantity can be done per round of practice.

Once the rhythm can be maintained and motion restricted to the abdomen, then you can begin a formal round of practice, which consists of 30 breaths in thirty seconds. Breathe normally for 2-3 breaths, and then repeat the process for a second round. You can do up to three rounds of 30 breaths each provided your abdominal rhythm is steady. After completion, sit quietly and observe the effects of the practice. Your inner vision may be drawn to focus on some spot. Allow your attention to be directed to what is a naturally arising point of concentration. Stay still for some time to allow the full benefits to unfold. Sit for at least 3 minutes or go straight into your meditation practice from here.

Benefits

Regular practice can create an aura of lightness and bring clarity to your mind. It acts like a brake to excessive mentation. On a physical level persistent practice is also renown for relieving respiratory conditions, colds, eyestrain, allergies and other conditions that may be influenced by changes of the seasons or the quality of mucous in the linings of the nasal and sinus passages.

Signs of Success in Pranayama

Training in Classical Yoga pranayama is rarely given because there are few competent masters available to train teachers. There are many variables in this process and it is not recommended to pursue practice except in a face to face, teacher to student training. For those who seek to learn pranayama from a book beware of the difficulties. It can be confusing, and potentially harmful when done improperly. There is a potential for weakening the immune system which in turn can prolong illness. One line I recollect frequently due to my own foolish behavior in trying to master pranayama without asking for his supervision follows.

Pranayama cannot be learned by toil,
Try however many times one may.
Strain, and pain, and surely weariness
Are the most one can hope to gain.
Guru Gita 53

The <u>Yoga Sutras</u> are clear in their elucidation of the process of pranayama and the experiences that are signposts of following the Classical Yoga Meditation path, step-by-step in the sequence cited as Patanjali's sutras. By the practice of following the previous three disciplines, Prana naturally begins to change from its ordinary course.

Like many Yogic texts, the <u>Yogayajnavalkya Samhita</u> is a treatise of questions by the consort/student of the Yogi who seeks to learn how to love Her consort/guru more fully through learning Yoga. Yogi Yajnavalkya in speaking to his wife Gargi says that "prana extends beyond the body by twelve units. Dear learned Gargi, know that Prana resides in your body." [116] For the normal human the body measures 96 units (called angulas or finger widths) and Prana is said to extend 12 units beyond the physical body. Hence the Pranic body altogether measures one hundred and eight units.

A similar text written by Krishnamacharya's 9th century ancestor, Nathamuni writes in his Yogarahasya sloka (verse) 58 that "the Prana Vayu (current) is normally scattered around the individual and if the Prana is brought closer to the body it indicates better life." [117] The outward spreading Prana is a sign of loosing Prana. Hence, for the Yogini, Prana is not extended beyond the body but is contained within the body. One definition of a yogi is someone whose Prana does not escape their body. One who masters Prana can deliberately send it outward to another for healing, but except for that, the Prana is held within the Yogini's skin through the mastery of pratyahara via Mudras. Indeed, the skin itself is a channel for the subtlest of the five subpranas, Vyana.

Desikachar's commentary on the previous sloka states "If the breathing rate is reduced, then the rotation of the chakras gets reduced. This will help in prolonging life, preventing and reducing disease." The final sutras of the <u>Yoga Sutras</u> (II, 51-53) on Pranayama mention how to extend the training to the highest level, called the fourth method. It is a naturally arising form of pran-ayama. By breaking the word into different syllables this meaning is to "extend the prana", whereas the previous <u>Yoga Sutras</u> (II, 49-50) are about prana-yama, referring to the disciplines of prana.

II, 51
In the fourth method
one's breath is extended
into the Divine Life Force
and prana
is felt permeating everywhere,
transcending the attention
given to either
external or internal objects.

II, 52
As a result
of this pran-ayama,
the veil obscuring the radiant
Supreme light of the inner Self
dissolves.

II, 53
And as a result,
the mind becomes fit
for the process of contemplation.

The natural pranayama of Patanjali is often spoken of in reverential tones as it is considered an offering or a prayer. Wherever the mind is directed gives the same experience of unity. It clears the mind of preconceptions and illusory impressions. Pranayama is the focus of the third chapter of the thirteenth century text <u>Vasistha Samhita</u>, the collection of verses attributed to the sage Vasistha.   He states
• Those who are purified by Pranayama, Reach the supreme goal. . .
• Pranayama is the savior for those who are drowned in the ocean of the trans-migratory world. [118]

Reference to the process of breath ceasing is also given in the fourteenth century <u>Hatha Yoga Pradipika</u>, in its second chapter.
• By stopping the prana through retention, the mind becomes free from all modifications.

By thus practicing this Yoga,
One achieves the stage of Raja Yoga (supreme union). [119]

XV. Ayurvedic Yoga Therapist

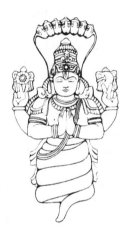

The Yoga Therapist's Role

The training of an Ayurvedic Yoga Therapist is the process of learning how to see the world through the Yogi's eyes. The Sanskrit word for this is Darshan (the way of seeing). Darshan implies both a way of seeing others and being an open window so that others begin to see the world through the expanded vision of the Yogini's perspective. The latter definition implies the ability to convey the experience of Classical Yoga, as a living breathing presence enlivened by prana Shakti. For such a profound opening to be available, the Yoga student must always remain a student of life. Learning how to accept and practice the integrity of the yamas and niyamas as a guideline toward an ethical lifestyle is crucial, much more important than the technicalities of philosophy, asana, pranayama and the variety of other Yogic discipline that are foundation for Yoga Therapy. Without this, the yoga community at large will not accept training and certification even if a respected teacher has given it.

The process of being a Yoga Therapist begins with your commitment to personal growth or in Sanskrit, sadhana. The word sadhana means literally "moving towards the Truth" or the "means to liberation." Attaining the Truth is a glimpse of liberation. Truth or satya is the second of the yogic code of ethics, the yamas. Satya - The words one says has the force of their life energy. When someone makes a commitment to class and then doesn't come or doesn't pay - where is the integrity in this action? With sufficient integrity the life energy of prana will manifest and words and actions will be mutually supportive. For details see <u>Yoga Sutras</u> II, 36.

The first principle in Yoga is nonviolence or ahimsa as cited in <u>Yoga Sutras</u> II, 33-35. The definition of nonviolence is the longest sutra (34) of the text; in summary it says, "negative thoughts and emotions are violent." In coming to class you bring with you your life force, your integrity. Those who are inspired and motivated naturally will come early, their intensity of searching for meaning in life is obvious. Look at yourself and see how you feel. When you feel good, your stamina, and energy level are elevated; when you feel bad your muscle strength goes down.

We know from Patanjali (<u>Yoga Sutras</u> II, 3-11) that for those students who identify with the body and are living on the path of sadhana, suffering is due to the influences of the five kleshas. The are ignorance of your True Self and the value of spirituality (avidya), egoism and its self centeredness (asmita), attachment to pleasure (raga), aversion to pain (dvesha), and clinging to life out of fear of death (abhinivesha). The process Patanjali recommends is to overcome them through meditation to reduce the reservoir of subliminal impressions that create karmic patterns. This involves being committed to moving through the layers of your personality defenses called the five koshas, so that the True Self can be revealed.

Each of the koshas can be seen as a defense mechanism that hides the True

Self. We are all born with a common physiology and psychology but the miracle of God's creativity is that we are absolutely unique. The manifestation of this lack of connection with spirituality and our True Self is the identification we have with our body and its instability. The instability is natural, in Ayurveda it is called the doshas, literally "that which is unstable." These seeds of instability sprout to manifest presence of fear, anger, and attachment as the imbalance of each of the doshas. According to Yoga philosophy in its attempts to explain our challenge, this instability arises out of a primal motivator called the gunas (sattva - balance, rajas - activity, and tamas - inactivity).

A primary objective of Yoga Therapy is to expand our capacity to be open, to revealing our True Self. This means being totally committed to the truth - in speech and action - supporting a life of integrity. The quality that is needed to facilitate this in others is a willingness to be fearlessly honest, first with yourself, and then with others.

This is a very difficult thing to do, and so it takes great courage. The truth is that we lie about a huge array of perceptions – the Truth of who we are, what we feel, what we want. This lying is a personal form of violence to the Self and from it arises a difficulty in sitting still with the Truth. Once this pattern of denying the truth is seen, we have the option of letting it go. Ignorance of the Truth, whether covert or overt, is stressful. Our goal is to get to the Truth, and then to help our clients get to their truth. In doing this, we can then begin to create change and help our clients create sattvic change.

A truthful person has no problem being still, holding to their words, their eyes show the stillness of the mountain pose. Good asana and pranayama practice can assist us in supporting the truth and living from that place in all our affairs. The Yogic perspective differs from the psychological one, in that the hidden agenda is not about any underlying hypocrisy but rather, that who we are is greater than we could imagine. By allowing ourselves to be vulnerable, we can move towards more clearly seeing who we truly are. The Yogi's agenda is to move beyond the koshas yet remain in this world, in our body, mind, and senses. We can experience the subtlest of the koshas as insightful illumination and as a seemingly endless stream of peace and love.

When we come from this place of understanding and compassion, can we be of help to others. The process of healing is the process of lifting the veils of mis-conception and misperception, elevating the doshas to their apex and allowing the pranas to evolve along their path to Self realization.

How to Work with a Client Using Ayurvedic based counseling

There is a primary role for therapists to take and there are secondary roles to assume. The prime directive of a Yoga Therapist is to be immovable like the consciousness of Shiva. That is, non-reactive and non-judgmental, while continually affirming the omnipresence of witness consciousness. This place exists as a gender neutral archetype within everyone. Yoginis learn it by doing sadhana and by being committed to personal growth as an eternal spiritual being having a human experience. From this arises clarity of what is permanent from direct experience. By having touched this consciousness even for a brief moment, they can be of true help to the client. What the client typically presents is an imbalance in the doshas and the gunas, and it is the Yoga Therapist's role to help the client move towards sattvic balance.

How does this happen? The Yoga Therapist must make a vow to themselves, under the guidance of their teacher, to live a lifestyle in alignment with the guidelines of Classical Yoga. This vow supports the intention to be of help to others. From this foundation your energy field will be in alignment and will serve to continually reveal new insights on how to manifest your vow.

Friend role for Vata

"Be sweet with Vata"

Just as there are three doshas, there can also be three different roles to take with working with each of the constitutionally predominant clients. Vata clients do best when the therapist takes the role of being their friend right from the beginning. This role can help them get over their discomfort at having a problem so they can reach effectively at resolving their hidden fears. These clients need a gentle approach, one that is built overtime and includes overcoming a series of small changes. They do best if they are not rushed into changes or even the feeling that you want them to change. Vata predominant client's motivation for change should come from within. In some cases they need to be perceived as a delicate flower needing plenty of comfort and patient attention for their flowering to blossom.

This constitution needs a role model. If they don't reveal one to you, then inquire until you find a person that they admire. They also need to be friendly and relaxed in order to reveal something of the tremendous fear and anxiety that they hold back from public display. It is OK to show something of yourself and of your struggles with life's challenges, but be careful to walk the delicate balance between therapist/ teacher and friend. Don't take them into your life; keep them separate from all personal involvements. They will tend to be secretive and if they see you not holding back something, their respect for the therapist will diminish. Once they see your friendliness is tinged with discernment then they will be appropriately secretive.

Once this is attained, then they will tend to retain their prana and be sattvic with you. This is often manifested as too soft, actually more of a tamasic quality, not ready for any real transformation. They change all the time, but rarely will they seek and commit themselves to a process of deep lasting transformation. This is what they want, yet it will take time to get all the elements of their preconceived ideas of a Yoga teacher/therapist intact before they will devote themselves to a program with you.

Spouse role for Pitta

"Be firm with Pitta"

Pitta predominant clients like and needs directness and a certain passion and enthusiasm. Here you are in the role assisting them, as you would your spouse, honestly conversing, evaluating and helping them to see the recommendations that they want to make. They do not seek advice easily and dislike being told what to do. Therefore, friendly questioning that guides the client to set goals and priorities of their own choosing, based on the information you help them perceive about themselves, allows them to feel more in control of their situation. Listen to their point of view including criticisms and judgments. Talk with them about any other practitioners they may have seen and be sure to ask them what they liked and didn't. Listen to what they have to say about other practitioners and be sure you to avoid those pitfalls. They may say, "he/she kept me waiting!" – then learn from this that they want you to be on time!

Pitta needs to be heard. When inflamed, they lose their perspective and their ability to discriminate, a hallmark of a balanced Pitta. They tend to be rajasic, over stimulating themselves with too much to do and not enough time to do it in. When they commit to something, they do it to the point of excess, aggravating themselves because they don't see the connection of doing a good thing too much. The motto of a Pitta unwilling or not ready to change might be heard as "If it is good then a lot of it is better."

A supportive, friendly spousal role will help them find their own discrimination and move to an innovative new direction.

Authority or Spiritual role for Kapha

"Show Kapha your stick"

Kapha needs to know that you know how to help them, that you have the necessary training, knowledge, and experience. They may or may not commit to you but if they do, it is because they see you as someone with depth of presence that can help them in a big way. Committing to their own work is less important to them than the fact that they trust you enough to recommend you to their closest friends. More than anything, they need to feel safe. They want to be challenged, even about their tendency to become lazy or sporadic in their efforts, but they need to feel consistently safe before you can challenge them.

Kapha predominant clients tend to be profoundly spiritual in their orientation to life but may not reveal it unless they have established a rapport with you. They are devoted in nature and, if spiritually evolving, are seeking where to place that loving, devotional quality so that it can be nurtured in an enduring connection with the Divine Presence. You might be their spiritual mentor if you are truly qualified by having a grounded spiritual practice and if they are seeking spirituality.

These clients will tend to be tamasic. They will not come regularly to appointments, or if they do, they will be late or they may call in sick at the last minute. By being friendly but firm with them, you will encourage them to respect you and to continue to work for a long period of time.

Teach what is within you,
Not as it applies to you, to yourself
But as it applies to the other.
It is not that the personal must accommodate himself to yoga
But rather that yoga must be tailored to suit each person.[120]

XVI. Overcoming Obstacles to Healing

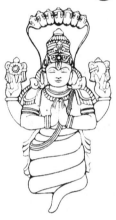

According to Patanjali's Yoga Sutras surrender to God overcomes all obstacles.

From that practice (of surrender to God)
arises attainment of inward directed consciousness
and also all the obstacles to successdisappear.[121]

Patanjali is a remarkable Yogi. He gives the highest technique before mentioning what it can do. You don't even have to know the obstacles, if you're doing that kind of practice. But the way Patanjali writes is that he pretty much raises an issue and then explains it. He continues to do that all the way through.

The Signs of Obstacles

According to the next sutra, number 30, the obstacles are those factors that "disrupt and scatter the mind." They are: disease. Second, dullness. Third, doubt. Fourth, negligence. Fifth, laziness. Sixth, dissipation, which results from excessive craving. Seventh, delusion. Eighth, lack of concentration necessary to achieve higher consciousness. The last one is instability.

The sincere Yogini is one in whom obstacles to healing on all levels simply arise from spiritual practice and their persistence allows them to fall away. One who spends time with a spiritual teacher or guru is that they tend to have more obstacles manifest than in the periods of being alone or with worldly people. By being around a teacher or a spiritual community both sides of the equation obstacles and their falling away due to devotion are heightened. The obstacles to devotion, physical and spiritual healing may feel like they are in your face, crowding one into a corner of the maze of life. As sadhana continues it often feels like these obstacles are pulled out by the roots. If you had doubts before, imagine a doubt as big as the house. If you had inconsistency, imagine being inconsistency such that you can't complete anything. You can't hold down a job, you can't hold down a relationship, you can't get to practice on time. Whatever your issue is, it gets blown up. That's one of the signs of a very good practice.

It's the same way with a lot of natural medicine. When you take the medicine, your symptoms increase before getting better, that's how yoga works too. It is how you know it is effective. Either the problem gets enormous or it simply vanishes.

Assessing for Obstacles with Breath and Pulse

Patanjali says that there are four preliminary indications of sickness that arise prior to the obstacles - distress, dejection, bodily restlessness and disturbed inhalation and exhalation. Four things. These are the first signs that a person is experiencing an imbalance in the doshas and pranas. One may not realize a person is having doubt or you might not get that a person is unstable unless you look for one of these four indications. One of the most important tools that I use to assess how sick or spiritually suffering my clients are is to look at their breathing and pulse. Is it steady or unsteady. When I feel the pulses, I ask clients to breathe more. The deeper breathing will bring out the latent tendencies of the pulse to show what is hidden subtly. For clients who don't have a spiritual practice, I don't do that because I'm not interested in subtle signs yet. But for a lot of people, I'll ask to read the pulse and read the breath so that I can tell from that reading where to take the therapy. It helps me to see where the opening is and what avenues are available for transformation.

I watch to see where the breath is naturally moving. For a lot of people, the breath is moving in the belly, not much in the chest. So that means that we can do an asana or pranayama practice and work with that opening. Different regions of the body are indicators of different types of prana, and I can also read the prana through the Ayurvedic doshas. If I'm reading through the prana and I see that your breath is active in the abdomen, then I know Samana (digestion) prana is active. It can be both mental and physical. When I see that, I know I need to go slowly with the person. I need to make sure they digest it, because I don't want to put too much physical/emotional/mental food in there. When you're taking something in there's a shift in the pranas. When you're digesting there is another shift. When you understand it, there's another shift. When you're letting go of the old information, there is yet another shift. When you've assimilated it, your aura gets bigger. There are 5 shifts, 5 pranas. I read this constantly while I'm watching and working with a client.

From Ayurveda, I use mostly the pulse to diagnose the Doshas: Vata, Pitta, Kapha pulses. Each of these pulses represents a different aspect: Vata, which is about the mind; the Pitta, which is about the vital energy; and Kapha, which is about the stability of the physical body and long-term health. The training of a Yoga Therapist is really about becoming extremely perceptive and understanding what the perception is that you are having. The signs are there and they're constantly available. Our sadhana is for the purpose of encouraging us to become more and more sensitive to the openings that change is revealing.

The pulses are reading the heart. They tell what's happening with the heart on several levels. You can read the physical heart organ and all of the other organs, or we can go down to a subtler pulse and read the heart energy. Moving to a subtler pulse yet, we get a sense of how that person might connect to spirit. Everyone will connect to spirit. But how? It's different from person to person. Beneath the surface, there is a phenomenal amount of activity going on. We all live in glass houses to someone who knows how to read. The details are unknown, but the general truths are very visible.

After reading the pulse and identifying what is needed, some clients with great self awareness can self adjust their pranas with minimum direction. Elizabeth's daughter is an example of this. She's someone that has a strong read for the truth, a remarkable young woman. She knew when the truth was being said and immediately shifted herself to follow that truth. Her energy was low and her pulse in the navel was off from where it should be. When the navel pulse is off center we lose energy; this is characteristic of people with autoimmune disorders especially when fatigue is a symptom.

A person with her strong Pitta predominant constitution should have an enormous amount of energy, but when I examined her she didn't. I said to her, I'm going to put your pulse back to center and she got it. As soon as I had her lie down on the floor to begin the exercises, I checked the pulse and she had centered it herself. I also found her sacrum was off. I said, since your mind is so strong you can do the same with your sacrum and told her how the sacrum should move to be in right position. She said, "Got it." I tested her. "Bingo." I didn't have to show her any adjustments, no exercises, nothing.

This is revealing strong indicators of an archetype student who will greatly benefit from the sadhana of the first chapter of Patanjali. They have to be shown the right way to go. They can change not only their body's function with their mind but also make dramatic life direction changes when they see the benefit in sound spiritual advice. For one whose mind is not adept at perception followed by discernment then taking appropriate action, Patanjali shows how to strengthen it, thereby increasing the ability to affect the changes desired.

Overcoming Obstacles with Yoga Discipline

Patanjali states, In order to prevent these obstacles from arising, one should habituate himself to meditation on a single principle. A list of meditation practices is given in sutras 34 through 39. Each of these sutras contains a technique you could stick to for the rest of your life if you chose to. Patanjali says that the ideal for meditation is to get a technique you really feel connected to and stick with it. For example, sutra 34 is a pranayama technique. It says that "to keep your mind serene is to forcibly exhale and retain the prana during the pause following the exhalation." Remember, when you exhale your belly should go in. If your belly doesn't go in, it will throw some things off. So practice exhaling and pulling back your central abdomen.

One technique is to concentrate on the fact that exhale goes in, pause, and then let the natural inhale come at its own time. Every time you exhale, make it with a mild, slight effort and then pause. Wait for the moment when it feels like you're ready to inhale, and then allow that to happen. Let it be completely natural.

Let the pause be a pause, not a holding of your breath. Then let the inhale follow that. During the pause, let your mind become extremely crisp and alert, and look in yourself for the feeling of prana as life force. Hold your mind on the idea of retaining that prana when you find it. Don't let it escape your body. Prana will direct your attention as to where the prana should be to feel at home. So as you continue, the prana is going to build and build.

The second step is a series of faster exhales. You can do any number, but I would not recommend more than 30. It's a good idea to keep it fairly gentle and easy, so that you don't hyperventilate. Simply do a number you can sustain and keep a regular pace. Be sure you end on the exhale, as the technique is to find the prana after the exhale. Sometimes the pause won't be there. Sometimes it will. Just do some recovery breaths until you feel ready to do it again. Sometimes I notice people force the inhalation. They just don't want there to be a pause.

Wait, until you feel that prana building in your body. Sometimes it moves around, but eventually prana will go to its home. When pranas go to their home, your mind automatically gets quiet. Peace is the result of balanced prana. Do this technique up to 5 rounds. If it's done well, you'll go into meditation. If you're really good, you will be able to go right into deep meditation without directing your thoughts; they will simply vanish.

It's a very good indication of how well your subtle energy is doing. By this technique, you can see it very easily. Pranayama is the subtlest and quickest way to get yourself back into balance.

Yoga Sutra II, 47 - When asana is acquired then there naturally follows a cessation of the movements of breath. There is a cessation of breathing - you're not breathing. When your mind is engaged, you're asking yourself - how long is this going to go on for? But when you're really having a true pranayama experience it goes on and on and there's no mind. You are completely indifferent, perhaps saying something like, "I'm watching this thing and I'm not breathing." The pause can be after the exhalation or inhalation, but it is safest to teach it following the exhalation because there are fewer side effects.

According to the Yoga Sutras II, 48 there are three ways to train the breath – "according to its place in your body, time and number." means either training to breathe into a specific part of your body, such as your heart, or going to timing such as six breaths in and out; or giving a specific duration for the exercise such as 27 times. The purpose of the training is to make the prana prolonged and subtle. With it the mind takes on the same characteristics. Overtime the pranayama training dissolves the self centeredness of the mind. Without this quality the mind becomes pure consciousness and stress free.

In the yogic tradition, "stress originates in two attitudes: "I am the doer" and "It is for me." These attitudes underlie avidya, the obstacles to clear perception, which Patanjali described as misapprehension, confused values, excessive attachments, unreasonable dislikes, and insecurity. And these in turn lead to troubling emotions expressed as desire, anger, possessiveness, self-delusion, arrogance, and envy.   In practice, the outcome is invariably dukha – the constraints upon our physical and mental life that lead to illness and discontent." [122]

XVII. Healing through Yoga and Ayurveda

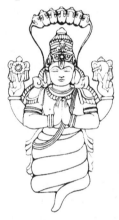

The classical text <u>Yoga Vasistha</u> has some intriguing points on healing and the interface of body and mind.

"Illnesses (vyadhi) and psychic disorders (adhi) are sources of sorrow. Their avoidance is happiness, their cessation is liberation. Sometimes they arise together, sometimes they cause each other and sometimes they follow each other. Both these are rooted in ignorance and wickedness. They end when self knowledge or knowledge of truth is attained." [123]

This quote points out the mental cause of disease interlaced with the resultant loss of happiness and discernment. When one is lost, the other factors are soon to follow. Emotional happiness and health are one and the same though we may perhaps see them as different dimensional aspects of the state of loss of health. This is a universal experience, as we can see from the following quote from a master healer of the Jewish tradition.

> "The basic cause of illness is unhappiness,
> and the great healer is joy."
> Rebbe Nachman of Breslov (1772-1810) [124]

We cannot cure ourselves of a malady unless we know what it means to be healthy. In the same respect we perceive directly when we are unhappy because intuitively we understand what happiness is. The great Jnana Yogi, Ramana Maharshi declared that "The desire for happiness is a proof of the ever-existent happiness of the (spiritual) Self. Otherwise how can desire for it arise? If headache were natural to human beings, no one would try to get rid of it. One desires only that which is natural to him: happiness, being natural, it is not acquired." [125]

This being the case, he said in his primal teachings of the path of self inquiry entitled Who am I? that "Since all living beings desire to be happy always, without any misery, since in everyone supreme love exists only for oneself, and since happiness alone is the cause of love, in order to obtain that happiness, which is one's very nature and which is experienced daily in deep sleep, where there is no mind, it is necessary for one to know oneself." [126] This is the highest teaching for the removal of all suffering regardless of where it is experienced as mental, physical, emotional or spiritual. The path of Self knowledge is for the removal of all suffering.

The <u>Yoga Vasistha</u> goes on to point out that "physical ailments are caused by ignorance and its concomitant total absence of mental restraint that leads to improper eating and living habits. Other causes are untimely and irregular activities, unhealthy habits, evil company, and wicked thoughts. They are also caused by the weakening of the nadi or by their being cluttered or clogged up, thus preventing the free flow of the life-force. Lastly, they are caused by unhealthy environment." [127]

These concepts form the foundation of what we call Natural Healing through maintenance of a healthy lifestyle. The previous quote shows that these contemporary concepts were well known in ancient history. Let us learn from the lessons of the past that we might lessen or expedite our healing today. By manifesting the Yogic lifestyle and incorporating Ayurvedic precepts, we can avoid or lessen the effects of illness and increase our mental and physical well being.

The overlap of Ayurvedic health care and Yogasana as sadhana is fairly extensive. "Medicine works on the body because it has a specific taste (rasa), quality (guna), potency (virya), effect (vipaka), and capacity (prabhava). Similarly, an asana has a perfect shape or correct formation (rasa), peculiar quality (guna), definite potency and intensity (virya), final resultant effect (vipaka), and specific nurturing capacity (prabhava). [128]

A Yogi's goal is similar yet different from that of an Ayurvedic physician. For the Ayurvedic doctor, the goal is to balance the doshas so that health may be maintained or restored. For the Yogi, the goal is to optimize health for the pursuit of Spiritual Liberation (moksha). More time is spent on spiritual practices than on health maintenance. I am not too concerned with the maintenance of health via balancing the doshas if in so doing one lessens the time and commitment to their spiritual sadhana.

A yoga student in England framed the question beautifully when he asked Yoga Master Desikachar "Did your father, Krishnamacharya, think that defects in the body are blockages which impair an individual's ability to move towards self realization?" Desikachar responded, "The very purpose of Yoga for him was to ensure that the body does not become an obstacle. That is the only reason for practicing Yoga and for maintaining health. If a person has perfect health, then why should he practice? So it was a step towards devotion. That's why when his own spiritual teacher became sick; my father (Krishnamacharya) became his Yoga teacher. The body should not become an obstacle for devotion. That is the only purpose for practicing health programs for the body." [129]

As a Yogi, I see all my clients as Yoga students whether they declare themselves to be or not. My goal is to enrich the foundational qualities of the balanced doshas. In this way their Vata quality will produce more sensitivity and intuition as to how pranic energy guides them. The goal for Pitta quality is to strengthen discernment so that they can know the mind as the source of spiritual light. For the Kapha quality, my goal is to encourage its qualities of compassion and open heartedness so that they can sustain more love and acceptance of themselves as they are. This ultimately will lead to the inner Self revealing its Presence.

An Ayurvedic practitioner may strive to increase the qualities that are opposite to the dosha qualities that have increased. The natural tendency is for your predominant constitutional quality to increase. So for a Kapha predominant client, they would recommend a Pitta increasing practice such as Ashtanga Yoga that heats the student and makes them sweat. In contrast, I strive to teach students to work with, rather than against, their predominant dosha. My idea is not to deny, lessen, or criticize it; but rather to seek a practice that brings attention to the dosha. When we focus our attention on the dosha (or any object of awareness), it will tend to increase (because prana increases from concentration); revealing its qualities more clearly. Then one can see what quality of the dosha needs emphasis in order to elevate it to a higher level.

In the case of Kapha, we want to direct attention to doing Yogasanas where we prolong the hold of the poses, thus bringing attention to the balanced state of Kapha - strength, stamina, open heart, humility and strive to enhance these qualities. As most seekers know, doing sadhana with sincerity and devotion can imbalance the doshas. The purpose of yoga is as a spiritual practice to remove the obstructive patterns laid down by years or even lifetimes of fixed mental attitudes and behaviors. The seeker is encouraged to develop a relationship with their body based on "consistent earnest effort and detachment from the results of that effort" as per Patanjali's recommendations for how to attain success (Yoga Sutras I, 12).

Kriya Yoga of the <u>*Yoga Sutras*</u>

Certainly one can utilize Yogasanas to help maintain balance in the unstable doshas, yet the Yogini as spiritual practitioner knows better than to put all their attention into only health. The concern for health is balanced with the need for purification, or Kriya Yoga. In chapter two of Patanjali's <u>Yoga Sutras</u>, Patanjali defines how to purify the mind through self discipline so that it can attain a higher level of consciousness capable of knowing the Self, which can lead to samadhi, regular periods of absorption in the Self.

Kriya Yoga consists of the first half of chapter two, sutras 1-28. The techniques of Kriya Yoga consist of self-study (swadhyaya), self-discipline and purification (tapas), and devotion to the Divine Presence (Isvarapranidhana). From following these guidelines as a practice rather than merely a philosophy, the student will evolve the three primal doshic qualities of biological and psychological functions. The yogic practices of self-study evolve the subtle air and ether qualities of Vata into Prana promoting greater perception, intuition and peace of mind. The practices of self-discipline and purification evolve the fire and water of Pitta into tejas giving the mind strength and the capacity for directing willpower into radiant discrimination. Similarly when devotion to "the Lord of your understanding" is sustained it produces humility and awareness of Oneness; this is the experience of ojas, created from the more fundamental quality of Kapha's earth and water. Once you understand and deeply connect with knowing yourself as love, there will be a movement towards living a life of increasing selfless service to others.

When these three qualities are balanced they naturally evolve from Vata to Pitta to Kapha. The practices that balance Vata and restore Prana will create the sensitivity that allows for Pitta to become balanced and generate tejas. This in turn sets up the conditions under which Kapha will evolve and create the nurturing substance of ojas. The cycle of balancing the doshas is Vata - Pitta - Kapha then back again, but now to a higher, more evolved Vata. The process of balancing the doshas tends to elevate their expression towards their essential nature as prana - tejas -

ojas. Thus as we work on improving ourselves through our daily practice of Yoga sadhana, our goal is to evolve our experience of ourselves into one of more loving kindness extended both to and from others and ourselves. On an emotional level this looks like Vata's imbalance as fear being overcome through faith and dissolving into it, resulting in knowing the truth directly. Pitta's judgment is transformed by inspiration into inspiration. Kapha's attachment to a personal truth is overcome by love until it becomes love.

The cycle begins with self observation (swadhyaya), sitting quietly and just looking at your current situation in life. By persisting in Self inquiry, insight will arise as the Prana rises.   When this Prana is fully developed it elicits a creative energy from the higher mind. A physical sign of this evolution is that your body relaxes in the lower abdomen and pelvic region. These are signs that Vata has returned home and is becoming balanced and evolving into Prana. Initially this can produce sensations of sexual arousal in some people, these sensations will relax with time and a deeper balance born of the sattvic state of Prana will develop. It is natural that any area where expression has been repressed will be senses as discomfort - until spiritual and mental health can find their personal expression.

A natural sign of this creativity is the arising of Pitta's energies of passion, vitality and the desire to freely act. There is an enthusiasm to share the vitality and joy that is natural to Pitta. For Pitta to fully evolve, the increased energy needs to be sustained until it creates a bodily reaction. For this to occur there must be a certain degree of regular discipline that consistently generates tejas. When this is sustained long enough, the abdomen, Pitta's home, becomes warm and softened. One sign of deep Pitta balance is that the central abdomen is felt to be the warmest part of the body.

This in turn gives one a feeling of satisfaction, natural to a healthy sign of Kapha, the heart is full and the righteousness of your actions is clear. Your mouth may literally become juicy, salivating with pleasure. When allowed to continue ojas will be born in the heart a sense of God's grace (Isvarapranidhana) will arise as gratefulness and gratitude pours over the soul, just from the pleasure of existing.

Evolution of the Vata – Pitta – Kapha Cycle

Into Self Inquiry

How do we begin this cycle? Inquiry into the Self. More specifically the question that evolves Vata into Self inquiry is - where is my energy? This can be emotional, physical, or subtle sensation that may not be recognizable with a particular label such as warmth, or fear, or hunger. Scan everywhere. By body scanning with the intention of simply finding the strongest sensations; you will begin to learn from your body kinesthesia. Do not try to label the sensations as that will distract you from learning from the raw experience. Merely look for the sensation, then place your hands there and give it your full attention. You might breathe into the area to give it more energy/awareness. Allow the currents of sensation to build until they captivate you.

When you are fully in the felt experience, then ask what the questions that will help Pitta to evolve – what does this energy want to do? Or where does this energy want to go? Let the energy build, again regardless of how it takes form. It may take the form of more thoughts, emotions, sensations, or intuitive insights. Keep repeating this process until there is a clarity that feels truly authentic. Do not rush. It is most important to uncover the Truth, not as you want it to be, but as it is. Begin to move with the increased energy, allowing the currents of sensation to physically express themselves no matter how it may look or feel. Continue to explore how to open yourself until there is a warmth and immediacy of presence in the motion.

When complete there is a feeling of resolution, and a naturally arising stillness. Then, the Kapha questions – "What will fulfill this desire/energy? What nurtures me?" - can be utilized until they generate the quality of ojas. The answer to wait for is a primal feeling of joy, which will arise naturally. Viewed from an Ayurvedic perspective, this deep joy occurs when the doshas are balanced. From a Yogic perspective, it arises of its own accord as the nature of the heart.

> One who is established in a comfortable posture
> while concentrating on the inner Self alone,
> naturally becomes immersed in the spontaneous
> arising of the Heart's ocean of bliss.
> Siva Sutras III, 16 [130]

In summary this path of inquiry is a bodily oriented series of questions based on looking at your energy body as the Spirit of guidance –

For evolving Vata - Where is my energy? Once you clearly locate it then ask.

For evolving Pitta - What does it want to do? And then do what your energy guides you to do.

For evolving Kapha - What takes me to completion? And finish what the energy has led you to until a deep stillness arises.

When this cycle is done there is a tremendous feeling of Prana. Pranayama is the balancing of the Pranic field within the body/mind complex that produces the awareness of Spirit. Open to each of these feelings, desires, and nurturing qualities and retain the gifts that arise from this meditation in your pelvis, belly and heart homes of the tridoshas.

Ayurvedic View of the Serenity Prayer

The Serenity Prayer is well known as the central offering of humility in the twelve step programs of recovery from addictive behavior and substances. It was given to Bill W., the co-founder of Alcoholics Anonymous, as part of the foundation for connecting to a Higher Power than yourself as a source for freedom from addiction.

God (Higher Power) grant me
the serenity to accept the things I cannot change,
courage to change the things I can,
and wisdom to know the difference.
Thy will, not mine, be done.[131]

From an Ayurvedic perspective, the Serenity Prayer is an expression of the culmination of the doshas balanced and elevated to their higher expressions. The experience of serenity is a lofty expansion of Vata as Prana comes home to bring the mind to its root of stillness. Courage is the natural expression of Kapha balanced then elevated to its higher mode as ojas, centered resting in the heart space. Wisdom is the experience of Pitta in its elevated state as tejas, which naturally produces insight, as the spiritual state unveiling the true nature of the mind as light.

When one is under stress, this prayer is very helpful for balancing all the doshas, if done repetitively with earnest seeking and surrendering to the Higher Power in whatever form you conceive that Presence to be in your life. Although I have never had the difficulty of alcoholism, I have personally found it to be of profound help during the most difficult periods of my life.

Yoga Pranic Healing

The popular contemporary concept of health as it relates to Yoga is defined in the principles of holistic health. The root origin of the word health is from the word whole. Whole health incorporates a full sense of well-being, mentally psychically, physically and spiritually. This fullness of health includes calmness and serenity, intuitive functions operating at peak capacity, physical well being with abundant energy for daily tasks and the unpredictable changes life brings, and a spiritual well being from knowing the creator and being in a relationship based in humility with their Higher Power as they conceive It to be.

"Health and happiness are often mentioned in the same breath, and maybe this is why: physiology and emotions are inseparable. I believe that happiness is our natural state, that bliss is hardwired. Only when our systems get blocked, shut down, and disarrayed, do we experience the mood disorders that add up to unhappiness in the extreme." [132] Taken all together, this can be considered the concept of holistic health or well-being.

For the Yogi, the concept of healing is rooted in the same process as the disciplines leading to self-realization. The Sanskrit word for health is swastha, which literally translated means "living in one's own Self." Thus, health and spirituality are interconnected from both the Yogic and Ayurvedic perspective. It is a return to the "wholeness of life" by reconnecting your sense of self to the whole. The difference is that the Yogi does not stop there, but looks at all of the aspects of personality, when made whole, leads to the fullness of the radiant light of the inner Self.

One such experience of this light is described in the classic Advaita (nondual) text of the <u>Astavakra Samhita.</u>

> Light is my very nature;
> I am no other than light.
> When the universe manifests itself,
> verily then, it is I that shine. [133]

In the same manner that one light manifests as the different colors of the spectrum when it becomes differentiated from its pure state, so also sound, feeling, taste and touch are also subdivided by the senses into distinct recognizable forms. While Pitta is the dosha that expresses light, the Ayurvedic subdosha referring to the primal quality of light is Pachaka Pitta. The Yogic concept of healing is based largely on the energies perceived through the second sheath, the pranamaya kosha, made of Prana. The quality of our Prana determines the quality of our physical, emotional and mental health.

The five Pranas function on a physiological level through the air element, but they function as emotions and subtle feelings as the ether element. To the Yogini, this energy is conceived as the breath but in a subtle dimension. Just as we can feel and see the effects of the wind without seeing wind, we can feel pranic effects without seeing prana. The Yogini can utilize the connection of breath and Prana to reintegrate with eternity. One definition of prana is "that which is infinitely everywhere."[134] This principle is the underlying characteristic of holistic healing. When we are healthy, we are healthy within our selves and our relationship to everyone and everything we encounter are healthy. When we are connected to the omnipresent, we are whole. When healing takes place, there is a reformation of the material world back to its primal elements.

Physicists tell us that the particles that make up the physical world including our body have been here since before the "Big Bang;" can we not also have faith in the truth of those Yoginis who gave gone before us stating their direct experience that prana is eternal? Where the two meet is in the common ground of the unexplainable, of mysticism.

One of my teachers taught that the world can be perceived on three levels. First, there is the known – that which we perceive with our mind and senses. The <u>Yoga Sutras</u> I, 7 describes the means of arriving at correct understanding from four sources – "direct perception, inference, revelation from reflections on the scriptures, or from the testimony of one who knows." [135] The second field of perception is the unknown - that which we may speculate on but have yet to comprehend but which can be known by directing our attention to seeking knowledge over a period of time. The third is the Unknowable - that which is not subject to perception by the mind and its constituent parts. By definition the last attribute of the world will always remain AS IT IS, unchangeable, infinite, yet Unknowable.

Experiencing Prana

How does one have a personal experience of this energy? A simple exercise to experience the body's prana can be done by rubbing your hands together until the friction creates heat in your palms. Separate your hands about a foot and bring them slowly close together until you experience something tangible yet non-physical between them. Gently move in and outward at the edge of this plane of energized space. If your sensitivity is elevated, you can also perform the same experiment by lightly touching your torso and slowly withdrawing from it. Focus your mind on the sensation that arises as your hands separate from your torso and as they come close together again. That tangible force felt around your body is Vyana Prana, commonly called the aura.

Swara Yoga - Yoga of the Breath Current

Another experiment to familiarize yourself with prana is to simply notice which nostril is most open. Take in a deep breath or close one nostril at a time and notice whether there is a difference between the nostrils. Sometimes you may perceive that both nostrils are evenly open, although it is more common for one or the other to be more open.

For the Yogi, this shows the pathway of a subtle form of prana that passes through nostril channels called the Ida and Pingala nadi. Ida means left, and Pingala means right, while nadi comes from the word nad meaning movement. The nostrils are the gross openings to subtle energy channels through which conscious awareness moves. When the nadis are closed, the individual experiences a dullness or inability to perceive, due to the predominance of the tamas guna. This form of Yoga practices aim at increasing openness in the channels to promote self-awareness and heightening sensitivity.

In the medieval period of Yogic literature, what is now practiced as physical or Hatha Yoga was done in a fashion to transform the three middle veils (koshas) composed of the subtle energy body. This transformation is called Tantra Yoga. The root tan means energy and tra means to transform. The root to the word Hatha is the two syllables ha and tha, meaning sun and moon. This refers to the Tantrik concept of the energy body possessing a polarity of right and left which flowed through the Ida and Pingala nadis. Thus by balancing the flow in the two nostrils, the mind could be refined into its subtle constituent components and more easily disciplined. Swara Yoga is the specific path that focuses upon this practice. Swara means the "sound of one's own breath." It is an ancient science that reveals how the movements of prana can be controlled by manipulation of the breath.

A subtler experiment is to observe which nostril is most open with your arms and legs first uncrossed, then crossed. You can also try this by interlacing your fingers. When the pranic channels are unobstructed by congestion from excess Kapha, the side that is on top will reveal the nostril that is dominant. That is if your right arm, finger, or leg is on top, then your right nostril will become more open and more breath will flow through. This change usually takes from 10-60 seconds, so if you didn't observe a difference wait longer and breath more deeply. What neurological mechanism makes this occur is not understood in terms of physiology. The Yogis focused their internal exploration experiments on reflexes that affected respiration and the sense of self and took advantage of them to alter their state of mind.

My last Hatha Yoga teacher, Indra Devi, was a master of this practice. Indra Devi was known as the "first woman of Yoga " as she was the first Western woman (from Latvia in northwest Russia) to be trained as a Yoga teacher by Krishnamacharya in 1937. Through his encouragement she spread yoga throughout the world.

"Yoga gives great importance to our relationship with the universe, and therefore it teaches a breathing that is different from the usual breathing, a breathing that reflects our inner attitude while we are performing it. This attitude is one of devotion, that is, of communion with the All, and should be maintained all the time one is doing deep breathing." [136]

Indra Devi believed that the alternating current was a living Presence that could be observed and cultivated to create an organic state of Yoga. She was adept at manipulating the pranic movements through her finger dexterity and often played finger games with me. She cautioned students not to cross their arms and legs (except at the ankles) as it interfered with the cosmic (Adya) Prana's ability to be received. She explained that by cultivating this awareness we would be more naturally open to others and to be blessed with the Presence of love and light that was the underlying reality of all life. She lived an extremely full life, passing away 3 weeks prior to her 103rd birthday in Buenos Aires, Argentina in April of 2002. Indeed I feel blessed in having her as my teacher over a 25 year period of my life.

Nostril predominance and brain hemisphere function have an opposite correlation. "Breath coming in through the right nostril cools the right hemisphere of the brain, causing the left hemisphere to become active. Breath coming in through the left nostril has the opposite effect." [137] The "right hemisphere of the brain is superior in terms of representational and visual spatial functions, in perception and discrimination of musical tones and speech intonations, in emotional responses, and in understanding humor and metaphor. In broad terms, the right hemisphere functions are holistic, spatial and hence are labeled 'artistic'. The left hemisphere is superior in motor and verbal skills, and appears to be specialized for logical and analytical operations; it categorizes things and reduces them to their parts in order to understand them. The right hemisphere is dominant in 97% of the population, while the left hemisphere is dominant in only 3%." [138]

Two of the methods used by Yogis to alter the predominant nostril current are the use of a Yoga Danda (a short crutch used as a sitting wooden staff) and lying on the side. Both of these methods take advantage of what I call the axillary reflex. [139]   This reflex, when stimulated by pressure on the upper chest wall in the armpit (axillary) region, causes "the breathing force to be increased in the nostril on the side opposite to the Yoga Danda and decreased in the nostril on the same side."[140] This is according to studies by Bhole and Karambelkar reported in the first journal of yoga physiology research "Yoga Mimamsa" dating to 1926.

The Yogis researched states of consciousness as they related to nostril dominance patterns and began to notice that one nostril dominance might be better suited for certain activities and emotional states. The shift in prana creates this nostril dominance called the Swara. Essentially the Swara shows which direction prana is beginning to flow. By observation of this change we can uncover whether or not our mind and actions are in harmony. The yogi's findings were recorded in texts such as the Shiva Swarodaya in a dialogue between Isvara and Devi (God and Goddess). "This knowledge of the Swara (current) is not merely for asking mundane questions. You should cultivate it for the sake of the Self (Atma). If you have the knowledge of Swara, it is not necessary to consult the date, stars, days, planets, gods, conjunction of the stars or disorders of the Ayurvedic dosha humors, before starting any project." [141] Shiva Swarodaya 28-29.

The text explains that left nostril breathing is sedative, so this is a time for meditation, sleep, spiritual practice and, for women having sexual relations. Often, by lying on the right side, the left nostril becomes dominant and it is easier to fall into a deep sleep this way. Right nostril dominance is stimulating, it is best for eating, hard physical work, purification practices and, for men, having sexual relations.

The implications of this phenomenon are that we are not victims of a given emotional state. We do have power to change our state of consciousness and emotionality. According to the principle researcher in this phenomenon, Dr. Shannahoff-Khalsa "If you want to alter an unwanted state, just breathe through the more congested nostril." [142]

There are three Swaras - one flows through the left nostril, another through the right, and the third when both nostrils are equally open. This third channel is known as the sushumna nadi. These three currents correspond to mind (chitta), life force (prana) and spirit (Kundalini or the atma), respectively. Mind controls the sensory nerves and organs. Prana controls the five organs of action – speech, hands, feet, reproductive and excretory organs. Spirit is the witness consciousness. As the breath flows through the alternating currents, a rhythm is created.

> "If the Swara (current) is irregular,
> it is a clear indication that something
> is not functioning properly in the body."[143]

Healing through the Five Pranas

Prana	location	motion	breath
Adya Prana	head, chest, heart	down & in	inhalation
Samana	small intestine	circular inward	pause after inhalation
Udana	throat, diaphragm	upward	1st phase of exhalation
Apana	large intestine	down & out	last phase of exhalation
Vyana	circulatory, lymph	diffusing outward	pause after exhale

There are many experiences of the five pranas. Some arise naturally from the increased sensitivity that comes from regular physical discipline. Some result from years of deliberate training under the guidance of a master in meditation or Yoga. Some dancers can also experience this; especially those who have learned to observe and participate in the greater dance that is within the human body. As one dancer described it -

"In the study of rhythm you can think of five main breaths.
Thinking of feeling the breath that rises
will lift you onto your toes with chest high.
Think of the breath that descends, and the chest is
forced down with the knees tending to give.
The breath that is horizontal will lead the body in full, round movements.
The breath that articulates is the breath you can
think of as being anywhere in the body.
The general breath is what we know as simple,
unconscious inhaling and exhaling." [144]

These five motions are a Divine Dancers experience of the five pranas -
- Udana - Apana - Samana - Vyana - Adya Prana, respectively.

Adya (Primary) Prana

The primary prana, Adya Prana, is formless, omnipresent and unchanging. This is the universal Prana that Desikachar defines as "that which is infinitely present." From the awareness of this energy one's consciousness gains a feeling of universal connectedness. In the individual, this subdosha of Vata is experienced in the body as coming downward and inward. "The prefix pra of the word prana means forward, toward or prior and relates to absorption." [145] It is commonly thought of as the movement of the inspiratory breath, yet it is not exactly that. More appropriately, it is the energy behind that motion, it comes first and the breath follows second. Like all pranas, it has many qualities; it can be balanced or imbalanced, excessive or diminished, moving home or displaced, pure or mixed with the features of other pranas. The very act of perceiving it, influences it. A state of acceptance and respect is central to helping someone heal. Allowing neutrality that comes from detachment to a specific outcome, increases the Adya Prana. Nurturance increases the Adya Prana.

Healers have this energy consistently. They don't need to obtain it from some place outside the Self; in fact it increases by expanding our perspective of what it is. By remembering the Tantrik experiential concept that what is outside is also inside, healing can happen spontaneously and naturally. The healing that happens through this prana is the most unexpected and unpredictable, because it comes from a place beyond mind - and even beyond good intentions. Health and well-being are natural states of Adya Prana, and the Yogi as healer, accepts whatever comes.

The Adya Prana governs respiration in general and inspiration specifically; it also regulates our capacity for intake in general, especially for sensory and intellectual information. When we stop listening to the message that Adya Prana gives us, we experience stress. From the pranic point of view, illness is due to ignoring the advice of the messages that the pranas are constantly sending. As we observe our pranas we can see what the inner teacher is seeking to enhance or lessen. When digesting food samana prana is likely to be active, but if we do not listen to this prana and engage in physical exertion then the prana becomes corrupted and as a result Adya Prana diminishes. Then we cannot take in the instruction of what we are seeking to do in our physical activity. As a result of this inattentiveness we may become careless and then injured.

Samana Prana

The second prana is Samana Prana. Samana means "to breathe together" from the roots "sam" meaning together and "na" meaning to breathe, or "equalizing air" from the root sama meaning "same." It predominates during the pause that follows the inspiratory motion of Adya Prana. It forms a circular pattern, spreading outward from the central abdomen to the upper right side across the upper abdomen then down the left side towards the pelvis. Thus it follows the path of the colon or large intestine. This prana's primary function is to receive nourishment by aiding digestion. This prana is related to Pitta's quality of discernment. When Samana Prana is healthy we can discern what is beneficial and allow it to come in. Thus, it governs digestion on all dimensions. It helps us to digest what we have received through the Adya Prana into the five senses, whether it is food, visual imagery, music, or physical touch. Samana Prana is also predominant in the arterial circulatory system as it spreads outward to all the tissues and cells.

Udana Prana

The third prana is Udana Prana or "upward moving" prana. It is the initial upward motion of the exhalation from the abdominal cavity. Its direction and force are opposite to the Adya Prana. It is the force through which excess Kapha is best expelled, up and outward through the orifices of the head. When it is functioning well, we discharge what is not beneficial and what is unwanted. It can generate feelings of happiness and lightness. Though when it is in excess it makes us light headed, dizzy, and disoriented.

When Udana Prana is evolved to a higher dimension of self, it propels spiritual awakening. It is then called Kundalini, meaning "coiled serpent". During quickening of Spirit, the serpent like force uncoils from its resting place and moves in the subtle body channel of the sushumna nadi, clearing out memories, impressions, attitudes, and suppressed emotions that are no longer beneficial. Though Kundalini awakening is not directly spoken of in the Yoga Sutras, the spiritual purification process is referred to in a general manner in the first portion of the second chapter of the Yoga Sutras as the Kriya Yoga cited earlier.

It is best to move into the experience of Udana Prana as a spiritual force with the support of a spiritual community or an experienced spiritual teacher. This is because spiritual awakening can be confusing or disorienting when compared to what one hears in superficial conversation or reads from books. Each spiritual path is different and what characterizes a beneficial purification to one group is seen as a potentially harmful practice to another group. Otherwise spiritual awakening can easily be misunderstood for the awesome gift of Grace that it truly is.

Apana Prana

The fourth prana, Apana, comes at the end of the exhalation. Apana refers to the "downward moving" prana. It promotes a feeling of acceptance and relaxation in the lower abdomen and pelvis. Its primary motion is downward and outward, and it is the force behind the expulsion of excessive Pitta and Vata. When Apana prana is unhealthy, these imbalanced doshas can cause problems in the site where they are obstructed and excessive.

Apana's primary function is to remove waste material from the body through the pelvic orifices. It is the energy behind urination and defecation. In women, it is the force pushing the menstrual fluid and the fetus from the uterus. I have experienced guiding a friend in the cultivation of her Apana Prana on the last night of her pregnancy. She was 43 and was having her first and only child as a single mother from artificial insemination. I taught her to lengthen the exhalation and relax her lower abdomen and pelvic region (the home site of Apana Prana). For 8 hours she was experiencing ecstatic waves of Adya and Udana Pranic energy moving downward and upward through her body. These waves generated a host of ecstatic experiences that included repetitive orgasms, visions of Kundalini's primal quality as radiant light, and insights into how she could let more friends into her life to assist her at learning motherhood. She very exuberantly told me that this was the most joy and happiness that she had ever experienced in her life. Finally at 6 am she felt Daniel ready to come out of her uterus. She delivered within an hour of her arrival at the hospital.

Vyana Prana

The fifth and final prana is Vyana, "vi" means "apart or to separate," and is the subtle energy during the pause following natural exhalation. It spreads outward in a circular motion opposite to that of Samana prana, except its spiral moves inward while Samana spirals outward. It functions as venous circulation and on the psychic realm we experience it as our aura, a protective bubble that keeps us safe from harm. This Prana is often felt as a protective force warning us when danger is near or to warn us when we are in questionable situations. It is through this prana that we dream, travel in space and time, and have out-of-the-body experiences. When evolved, Vyana Prana is a doorway to meditation and ultimately to the continuous awareness of the True Self. One method taught by Patanjali for the evolution of this prana is given in his Yoga Sutras I, 34.

> Or another way to lessen the obstacles
> and keep the mind serene
> is to forcibly exhale
> then retain the prana
> during the pause
> following the exhalation.[146]

By this practice, the Apana Prana becomes prominent and with it the pause becomes lengthened. Through that pause the presence of unity consciousness is more accessible.

Healing the Mind through the Doshas

The primary issues for which people enter psychotherapy can be framed from an Ayurvedic dosha viewpoint as fear, anger, and attachment. These are excess of Vata, Pitta, and Kapha respectively. Fear is Vata's twisted form of the search for peace. People challenged by this situation are described as 'tight assed', 'anxiety ridden', or as 'making mountains out of molehills'. When Vata is balanced, fear and anxiety become resolved and serenity is restored.

Anger is Pitta's twisted form of search for vitality. It is commonly described as the feeling of your 'guts tied up in a knot' or the need to strike out to protect yourself from perceived threat. When Pitta is harmonized, the intestines relax and peristalsis resumes producing all the drive and enthusiasm one could ever hope for.

Attachment is Kapha's twisted form of a search for love, abundance, and acceptance. People with this difficulty are said to be 'tight fisted', 'closed hearted', or as 'stuck in the mud'. When Kapha's attachments are resolved then it helps to promote solid, lasting relationships that are healthy, nurturing and loving. This extends both inwardly to tissue and organ relationships and outwardly into social relations.

"Whatever the individual soul experiences within in dreams on account of the Vata, Pitta, and Kapha, that he experiences outside too, and in that field his own organs of action function appropriately. When agitated or disturbed inside and outside, he experiences a little disturbance if the disturbance is slight, and he experiences equanimity if they are in a state of balance or equilibrium. . . When they are in a state of equilibrium, the jiva residing within them sees the whole world as it is, as it really IS, non-different from Brahman." [147]

The major emphasis on healing using Yoga techniques is keep the focus on your own sadhana as the most appropriate means to health. Returning to the Self is health. Only from healing yourself can the understanding of how to heal others emerge. As each of the doshas become refined they produce a quality that uplifts the mind making spiritual qualities more accessible. Vata produces prana that increases intuition. Pitta creates tejas that gives the experience of everything as light. Kapha produces ojas that gives both physical and mental endurance and persistence.

Apex of the Doshas - Prana, Tejas, Ojas

Through the process of balancing and evolving the doshas - Vata, Pitta, and Kapha - their subtle elements become generated. These are respectively called Prana, Tejas and Ojas. Together, these three are the composition of the subtle body. They are the matter behind Pranayama kosha, Manomaya kosha and Vijnanamaya kosha. Vata, Pitta, and Kapha; they relate to the gross functions of breath, digestion and physical health. The subtler essence relates to the soul's desire for Spirit, higher intelligence and devotion to the Source. It is the transformation that the Ayurvedic practitioner seeks through her/his cultivation of the life science. For the Yogi, these are naturally arising from doing elevated practices and being in the company of illuminated souls.

This form of Prana is different than those mentioned previously in the subdoshas. This Prana is the physical essence of Spirit as it manifests in the body. Prana evolves from the balance of the subtle functioning of the physiology and seeks to go beyond the identification of the self with the body. Prana promotes to the ordinary tissue and the mind's ability to adapt to change, also, contributing to creativity and the desire to evolve. Prana provides us with the desire to procreate, the will to live and sustain life. It is the breath of life imparted to the individual through live organic foods. This results in the feeling of connectedness to the cycle of life. In the mind, it manifest as peace.

From healthy Pitta, comes the fire of discernment that directs one toward good and creates indifference to that which is destructive. The being instinctively knows the difference between healthy and unhealthy activities and is able to make consistent choices for the betterment of themselves and those they serve. Tejas is the refined component of the Pitta dosha that particularly manifests in the Manomaya Kosha as intelligence and the ability to assimilate new information. Tejas is the light of consciousness whose source is the all-pervasive Self as Purusha. Tejas is the discriminative factor of the being that results from a spiritual illumination. It is the fire of higher intelligence that builds one's passions to know the truth of human existence. It is the one that asks, "Who am I?" and "Why am I here?" It manifests as the spiritual quest and the craving for living in the light of Spirit.

Ojas builds upon the foundation of a balanced Kapha, as physical and emotional strength and stamina, into creating a vibrant and healthy immune system. Ojas is the refinement of Kapha and manifests on all the bodies. For the physical body, it is expressed as the stamina of the immune system. Ojas in the pranic body, it is the vitality and vigor of the Life Force. In the mind it is joi de vie. In the wisdom body, it is the quest for an ever-deepening understanding and love of knowledge. In the bliss body, it is the loss of self and the bliss of the nature of the Self as perpetual, ever unfolding Love. This strength, stamina and health lead to an open heart. It is much more than physical health and the absence of pain. Ojas manifests physically as our sexual fluids and additionally in women, it is the life giving force of a mother's good heart becoming breast milk. Its fullest expression is love of all life.

These three forces are more interrelated than the tri-doshas. While it is true that an imbalanced Vata will lead to Pitta and Kapha derangements, an excess or diminishment of Prana, Tejas or Ojas will more immediately change the others. Low Ojas will tend to excite Prana and Tejas. While increased Prana tends to dry out Ojas, diminished Prana tends to decrease the flow of Ojas.

The Heart of Healing

The first chapter of the <u>Yoga Sutras</u> contains the practices for meditation and experiencing the Divine Presence. Patanjali begins with the highest teaching in the opening sutra:

"With great respect and love
now the blessings of
Yoga instruction can be offered."[148]

That's the key for profound healing. Developing your qualities of respect and love, and cultivating the goodness of your own Heart allows humility to come forth. This must be developed before one can be a Yogi or a healer. If one doesn't come from that place, they're not going to be very successful at experiencing Yoga's depth. The first sutra's message is that you have to come from that place of "great respect and love" in order to both give and receive the teachings. If we're in a place of respect and openness and our attitude is open and available to serve, we don't need instruction in asana, and don't even have to be told about chakras and subtle energy fields, because we're wide open. But if we're not at that level, we have to learn these things and that is the curriculum for the second archetypal student in Patanjali's systematic teachings, which is cited in the second chapter.

You don't need to ask how to cultivate openness. You are naturally open and receptive to life. You go around with the attitude, "God is within all life and That One is going to teach me; what can I learn?," and you are automatically drawn to very, very high teachers. You are pulled to teachers who can move you ahead and are indifferent to teachers who are inappropriate for you.

Ayurvedic Yoga Therapy Approach to Disease

The scope of Ayurvedic medicine is equivalent to Internal Medicine yet it goes beyond what we consider Allopathic Internal Medicine to be in that it incorporates a holistic perspective. The definition of Ayurveda is given in the medical textbook Caraka Samhita, Sutrasthanam I, 41-42 as "that science is designated as Ayurveda where advantageous and disadvantageous as well as happy and unhappy states of life along with what is good and bad for life, its measurement and life itself are described. The term 'ayus' stands for the combination of the body, sense organs, mind and soul, and it synonyms are dhari (the one that prevents the body from decay), jivita (which maintains life), nityaga which serves as a permanent substratum of this body) and anubandha (which transmigrates from one body to another)." [149]

In India, Ayurvedic physicians are trained to maintain health through the recommendation of beneficial activities for diet, use of herbs, lifestyle, family planning, and even the satisfaction of natural urges with aphrodisiacs.[150] This is meant to assist the individual in fulfilling the four goals of life - righteous duties (dharma), appropriate financial abundance (artha), sensual pleasure (kama), and spiritual liberation (moksha).

The Yogi seeks to utilize basic Ayurvedic principles help to cultivate and maintain a healthy disciplined lifestyle focused on spiritual fulfillment and ultimately realization. The Yogi is more like the minister who is more focused on your soul's evolution than your physical health. Of course a highly evolved person will be empathetic to all your concerns, and may have a broader based competency for dealing with them.

Krishnamacharya's ancestor from the 9th century, Nathamuni composed a text called the Yogarahasya. It contains some intriguing comments on integrating concerns for health and healing.

"For earning a livelihood or for the service of God, good health and a strong body are absolutely essential.

A person with disease, whether rich or poor, a king or a scholar can never have mental quietude.

Some diseases are cured by asana practice, some by pranayama, some by regulated diet and some by meditation. And some diseases are cured by religious activities.

When the body is diseased use asana practice to cure; when the mind is disturbed, make use of the techniques of pranayama.

When medicines cannot remove a disease, then definitely, the proper practice of yoga will help.

To cure many types of diseases, many different techniques have to be tried and adapted. However asana practice must always be accompanied by regulation of the breath." [151]

XVIII. Footnotes

1 David Frawley. <u>Yoga and Ayurveda</u>. Twin Lakes, WI: Lotus Press, 1999, preface, page iii.

2 David Frawley and Sandra Summerfield Kozak. <u>Yoga for Your Type.</u> Twin Lakes, WI: Lotus Press, 2001, pg. 11.

3 There are several texts that speak of this. Among them is the introductory sloka to the <u>Guru Gita</u>.

4 <u>Caraka Samhita</u>, op. cit., pg. 40.

5 <u>Ibid</u>. Yoga Sutras II, 2.

6 Vasant Lad. <u>Ayurveda – the Science of Self-Healing</u>. Wilmot, WI: Lotus Press, 1985, pg. 31.

7 Mukunda Stiles. <u>Yoga Sutras of Patanjali</u>. Boston: Weiser, 2002, pg. 30.

8 Ram Karan Sharma and Vaidya Bhagwan Dash. <u>Agnivesa's Caraka Samhita</u>. Varanasi: Chowkhamba Sanskrit Series Office, 1976, pg. 43, Sutrastanam I, 59-61 states that an increase in the doshas is "reconciled by medicines having opposite qualities.

9 Mukunda Stiles. <u>Yoga Sutras of Patanjali</u>. Boston: Weiser, 2002, pg. 26.

10 Mukunda Stiles. <u>Yoga Sutras of Patanjali</u>. Boston: Weiser, 2002, pg. xx.

11 Gabriel Cousens, MD. <u>Spiritual Nutrition and the Rainbow Diet.</u> Boulder, CO: Cassandra Press, 1986, pg. 115.

12 During an evening program Aug. 20, 1981 at SYDA ashram in South Fallsburg, NY.

13 Quoted on MS Society T-shirt fund raiser.

14 William Chittick. <u>The Sufi Path of Love: The Spiritual Teachings of Rumi</u>. Albany: State University of New York Press, 1983, pg. 238-239.

15 To determine your individual constitution, I recommend you read <u>Prakruti - Your Ayurvedic Constitution</u> by Dr. Robert Svoboda. Albuquerque, NM: Geocom Limited, 1989. This book gives sound advice for self-diagnosis and recommendations to restore balance by the only American trained as a full Ayurvedic physician.

16 My "magic bullet" is described as the sacroiliac stabilizing exercise on the archival website containing over 200 pages of my answers to questions students have raised on Yoga Therapy. Go to www.yogaforums.com and search by topic for details.

17 Mukunda Stiles. <u>Yoga Sutras of Patanjali</u>. Boston: Red Wheel/Weiser, 2002, pg. 25.

18 <u>The Nectar of Chanting.</u> Oakland, CA: SYDA Foundation, 1978, pg. 18 - <u>Guru Gita</u>, last introductory mantra.

19 Mukunda Stiles. <u>Yoga Sutras of Patanjali.</u> Boston: Weiser Books, 2002, pg. xvi.

20 Mukunda Stiles. <u>Yoga Sutras of Patanjali.</u> Boston: Weiser Books, 2002, pg. 16.

21 Mukunda Stiles. <u>Structural Yoga Therapy</u>. York Beach, ME: Samuel Weiser, Inc., 2000, pgs. 7-8.

[22] 5 Desikachar, T. K. V. with R. H. Cravens. Health, Healing & Beyond – Yoga & The Living Tradition of Krishnamacharya. New York: Aperture, 1998, pg. 61

[23] For a good overview of how to personalize Ayurveda see Robert Svoboda's Prakruti – Your Ayurvedic Constitution. For a more in-depth study see David Frawley's Ayurvedic Healing.

[24] Ramana Maharshi (1879-1950) is one of India's greatest sages. His teachings are the apex of Yoga and are summarized in The Spiritual Teachings of Ramana Maharshi, with an introduction by Carl Jung. A catalog of books, videos, and a free bi-monthly newsletter are available at Ashrama@aol.com or call 718-575-3215.

[25] See recommended readings.

[26] C. Mackenzie Brown. The Song of the Goddess – The Devi Gita. Albany: SUNY Press, 2002, back cover.

[27] John Douillard. The 3-Season Diet. New York: Harmony Books, 2000.

[28] Ram Karan Sharma and Vaidya Bhagwan Dash. Agnivesa's Caraka Samhita. Varanasi: Chowkhamba Sanskrit Series Office, 1976, pg. 146, see Sutrasthana VII, 3-5.

[29] Ibid., pg. 150-151, Sutrasthana VII, 26-30.

[30] Mukunda Stiles. Yoga Sutras of Patanjali. Boston: Weiser, 2002, pg. 24.

[31] "How to Tell when Someone's Lying". Tim Clark. Dublin, NH: The Old Farmer's Almanac, 2003, pg. 206.

[32] Mukunda Stiles. Yoga Sutras of Patanjali. Boston: Weiser, 2002, pg. 24.

[33] Srivatsa Ramaswami. Yoga for the Three Stages of Life. Rochester, VT: Inner Traditions, 2000, pg. 54.

[34] Swami Muktananda Paramahansa. Bhagawan Nityananda of Ganeshpuri. SYDA Foundation, S. Fallsburg, NY, 1996, pg. 130.

[35] The Nectar of Chanting, SYDA Foundation, Oakland, Ca., 1975, pg. 86.

[36] Paramahansa Yogananda. God Talks with Arjuna. The Bhagavad Gita II, 62-63. Los Angeles: Self-Realization Fellowship, 1995, Chapters 1-5, pg. 307.

[37] Paramahansa Yogananda. God Talks with Arjuna. The Bhagavad Gita IV, 38, pg. 521.

[38] Gheranda Samhita V, 16 and 22

[39] Bhagavad Gita XVII, 8-10

[40] Chandogya Upanishad VII, 26.2

[41] Swami Dayananda with Janaki Vunderink. Hatha Yoga for Meditators. South Fallsburg, NY: SYDA Foundation, 1981, pg. 110.

[42] Johanna Dwyer. "Health Aspects of a Vegetarian Diet", American Journal of Clinical Nutrition, 1988, 48: 712-738.

[43] Ram Karan Sharma and Vaidya Bhagwan Dash. Agnivesa's Caraka Samhita. Varanasi: Chowkhamba Sanskrit Series Office, 1976, pg. 46, see Sutrasthana I, 65..

[44] John Hole Jr. Human Anatomy and Physiology. Dubuque, Iowa: Wm. C. Brown Company Publishers, 1978, pg. 332.

[45] Wynn Kapit, Robert Macey, Esmail Meisami. The Physiology Coloring Book. NY: HarperCollins Publishers, 1987, pg. 98.

[46] Arthur Guyton. <u>Physiology of the Human Body</u>. NY: Saunders College Publishing, 1984, pg. 248.

[47] John Douillard. <u>Ayurvedic Pulse Reading Course.</u> Boulder, CO: lifespa.com, 1998, pg. 22. See also his excellent book <u>The 3-Season Diet</u>. NY: Harmony Books, 2000.

[48] Theos Bernard. <u>Hatha Yoga.</u> York Beach, Me: Samuel Weiser, 1972, page 47.

[49] <u>Hatha Yoga Pradipika</u>II, 31-32. commentary by Swami Muktibodhananda. Bihar, India: yoga Publications Trust, 2000, pg. 208-212.

[50] <u>Hatha Yoga Pradipika</u>II, 31-32. commentary by Swami Muktibodhananda. Bihar, India: yoga Publications Trust, 2000, pg. 206.

[51] Dr. RS Agarwal. <u>Secrets of Indian Medicine</u>. Pondicherry, India: Sri Aurobindo Ashram, l983, pg. 139. See also <u>Yoga of Perfect Eyesight,</u> by the same author.

[52] Sharma, Ram Karan and Vaidya Bhagwan Dash. <u>Agnivesa's Caraka Samhita</u>. Vol. 1 Sutra Sthana. Varanasi: Chowkhamba Sanskrit Series Office, 1976, pg. 151-153.

[53] Robert Svoboda. <u>Prakruti - Your Ayurvedic Constitution</u>. Albuquerque, Geocom Limited, 1989, pg. 107.

[54] Robert Svoboda. <u>Prakruti - Your Ayurvedic Constitution</u>. Albuquerque, Geocom Limited, 1989, pg. 110.

[55] Mukunda Stiles. <u>Yoga Sutras of Patanjali</u>. Boston: Weiser Books, 2002, pg. 28-29.

[56] Benson, Herbert. <u>The Relaxation Response</u>. NY: Avon Books, 1975.

[57] Mukunda Stiles. <u>Structural Yoga Therapy.</u> Boston: Redwheel/Weiser, Pg. 254.

[58] Frawley, David and Kozak, Sandra Summerfield. <u>Yoga for Your Type</u>. Twin Lakes, WI: Lotus Press, 2001.

[59] Geeta Iyengar. "Yoga and Ayurveda", Yoga '87. San Francisco: Iyengar Yoga Conference magazine, pg. 46.

[60] <u>Ibid.</u> pg. 43.

[61] TKV Desikachar. University of San Francisco lecture, Sept. 1980.

[62] Yogacarya T. Krishnamacharya. <u>Sri Nathamuni's Yogarahasya</u>. Translation by TKV Desikachar. Chennai: Krishnamacharya Yoga Mandiram, 1998, pg. 40, sloka 33.

[63] <u>Ibid</u>. pg. 46, sloka 45.

[64] Bass C. and Gardner W. Emotional influences on breathing and breathlessness. Journal of Psychosomatic Respiration 1985; 29: 599-609. also see Feleky A. The influence of the emotions on respiration. Journal of Exp. Psychology 1916; 1:218-241

[65] Susana Bloch, Madeleine Lemeignan and Nancy Aguilera-T. "Specific respiratory patterns distinguish among human basic emotions". International Journal of Psychophysiology, 11 (1991), pg. 141.

[66] Kirin Narayan. <u>Storytellers, Saints, and Scoundrels</u>. Philadelphia: University of Pennsylvania Press, 1989. (A sociology thesis on Swami Prakashananda and Hindu religious teaching). Titus Foster. See also <u>Agaram Bagaram Baba - Life, Teachings, and Parables -A Spiritual Biography of Baba Prakashananda</u>. Berkeley: North Atlantic Books and Patagonia, AZ: Essene Vision Books, 1999.

[67] Swami Prakashananda retells many of Muktananda's stories. <u>Don't Think of a Monkey and Other Stories my Guru Told Me.</u> Fremont: CA: Sarasvati Productions, 1994. (Note – this author is a different Swami Prakashananda, an American disciple of Swami Muktananda).

[68] MJN Smith. An Illustrated Guide to Asanas and Pranayama. Madras: Krishnamacharya Yoga Mandiram, 1980, pg. 14.

[69] Swami Venkatesananda, translator. <u>Vasistha's Yoga.</u> NY: SUNY Press, 1993, pg. 534.

[70] Paul Copeland. <u>Beginning Yoga with Narayana.</u> Davis, CA: unpublished manuscript, 1973, pg. 1. MJN Smith. <u>An Illustrated Guide to Asanas and Pranayama.</u> Madras: Krishnamacharya Yoga Mandiram, 1980, pg. 193. Also Gary Kraftsow. <u>Yoga of Wellness.</u> NY: Penguin, 1999, pg. 328.

[71] <u>Talks with Sri Ramana Maharshi.</u> Tiruvannamalai: India, 1994, pg. 106.

[72] Swami Nikhilananda. <u>The Upanishads.</u> Volume four. New York: Ramakrishna-Vivekananda Center, 1978, page 314-314.

[73] Robert Bly. <u>The Kabir Book.</u> Boston: Beacon Press, 1977, page 17.

[74] "Apa Bane, the Saint with the "Palm Disease", Ernst Feldtkeller. AS News – Journal of the National Ankylosing Spondylitis Society, East Sussex, UK, autumn/winter 2000, pgs. 8-10.

[75] Mukunda Stiles. <u>Yoga Sutras of Patanjali.</u> Boston: Red Wheel/Weiser, 2002, pg. 23.

[76] Swami Venkatesananda, translator. <u>Vasistha's Yoga. NY: SUNY, 1993, pg. 547.</u>

[77] Adapted from <u>Stories Retold</u> by Vijayendra Pratap in SKYwriting newsletter, Philadelphia: SKY Foundation, April 1993, page 1.

[78] Swami Venkatesananda. <u>The Concise Yoga Vasistha.</u> Albany: SUNY Press, 1984, pg. 140.

[79] Swami Muktibodhananda. <u>Hatha Yoga Pradipika.</u> Bihar, India: Yoga Publications Trust, 2000, pg. 132.

[80] Swami Satchitananda. <u>Integral Yoga Hatha.</u> New York: Holt, Rinehart, and Winston, 1970, pg. 25.

[81] Bhanawanvo Pant Pratinidhi (the Raja of Aundh). <u>Surya Namaskara - an Ancient Indian Exercise</u> – Hyderabad, Orient Longman, 1989.
Swami Satyananda. <u>Surya Namaskara (A Technique of Solar Vitalization).</u> Bihar: Bihar School of Yoga, 1983.

[82] Robert Svoboda. <u>Prakruti - Your Ayurvedic Constitution.</u> Albuquerque, Geocom Limited, 1989, pg. 110 – 111.

[83] John Douillard. <u>Body, Mind, and Sport.</u> New York: Crown Trade Paperbacks, 1994, pg. 198.

[84] <u>Ibid.</u>, 1994, pg. 183.

[85] Normandi Ellis. <u>Awakening Osiris: A New Translation of the Egyptian Book of the Dead.</u> Phanes Press, 1988, page 168.

[86] Michel Peissel. <u>Tibet - The Secret Continent.</u> London: Cassell Illustrated, 2002, pg. 42.

[87] <u>Rumi - We are Three.</u> Translated by Coleman Barks. Maypop Books, 1987, pages 20-21.

[88] This story is from Kalidasa's poem Kumara Sambhava (The Birth of the War Lord) and is adapted from commentaries by BKS Iyengar in Light on Yoga. New York: Schocken Books, 1979, pg. 69-70) and Margaret Stutley in her Illustrated Dictionary of Hindu Iconography. London: Routledge and Kegan Paul, l985, pg. 159.

[89] Jacqueline Decter. Nicholas Roerich – The Life and Art of a Russian Master. Rochester, VT: Park Street Press, 1989, dust jacket cover.

[90] Ibid, pg. 159.

[91] His Holiness the 14th Dalai Lama Southern Florida 2004 Program Guide, pg. 25.

[92] Baba Hari Dass. Ashtanga Yoga Primer. Santa Cruz, CA: Hanuman Fellowship, l976, pg. 11.

[93] Mukunda Stiles. Structural Yoga Therapy. Boston: Red Wheel/Weiser, 2001.

[94] Arthur Klein and Dava Sobel. Backache Relief. NY: Times Books, 1985, pages 79-81.

[95] Swami Digambaraji, editor. Hathapradipika of Svatmarama. Pune: Kaivalyadhama, SMYM Samiti, 1998, pg. 179. This is the only edition of this classic text to contain the fifth chapter.

[96] Ibid. pg. 180.

[97] Sadashiv Nimbalkar. Yoga for Health and Peace. Bombay: Yoga Vidya Niketan, 1985, pg. 316.

[98] Mukunda Stiles. Yoga Sutras of Patanjali. Boston: Red Wheel/Weiser, 2002, pg. 29 (II, 51).

[99] Mukunda Stiles. Yoga Sutras of Patanjali. Boston: Red Wheel/Weiser, 2002, pg. 28 (II, 46-47).

[100] A most helpful book in this regard is David Frawley's Tantric Yoga and the Wisdom Goddesses. Salt Lake City: Passage Press, 1996.

[101] Paul Eduardo Muller-Ortega. The Triadic Heart of Siva. Albany: SUNY Press, 1989, pg. 52-54.

[102] Mukunda Stiles. Yoga Sutras of Patanjali. Boston: Weiser, 2002, pg. 41.

[103] Richard C. Miller. Infinite Awakening. Workbook for Learning the Principles and Practice of Yoga Nidra. Sebastopol, CA: author, pg. 11.

NEW[104] Among the finest are Frank H. Netter, MD. Atlas of Human Anatomy. Summit, NJ: CIBA-GEIGY Corporation, 1996 and Carmine Clemente. Anatomy: A Regional Atlas of the Human Body. Philadelphia: Lea and Febiger, 1987.

[105] John Douillard. Body, Mind and Sport. NY: Crown Trade Paperbacks, 1994, pg. 165.

[106] Mukunda Stiles. Yoga Sutras of Patanjali. Boston: Weiser, 2002, pg. 29.

[107] Mukunda Stiles. Yoga Sutras of Patanjali. Boston: Red Wheel/Weiser, 2002, pg. 29

[108] Hathapradipika of Svatmarama. Swami Digambaraji and Pt. Raghunatha Kokaje, editors. Pune, India: Kaivalyadhama, 1998, pg. 183 and 188. NOTE – This is the only edition in print of this classical text that contains the fifth chapter.

[109] TKV Desikachar. Health, Healing & Beyond. NY: Aperture, 1998, pg. 107.

[110] Daniel Odier. Yoga Spandakarika – The Sacred Texts at the Origin of Tantra. Rochester, VT: Inner Traditions, 2005, pg. 150.

[111] Hathayoga Pradipika I, 55

[112] M.J.N. Smith An Illustrated Guide to Asanas and Pranayama. Madras: Krishnamacharya Yoga Mandiram, 1980, pg. 3.

[113] Swami Muktibodhananda Saraswati. Hatha Yoga Pradipika. Munger, India: Bihar School of Yoga, 1985, pg. 177 (Chapter II, 5).

[114] Mukunda Stiles. Structural Yoga Therapy. Boston: Weiser, 2000, page 145.

[115] Swami Muktibodhananda Saraswati. Hatha Yoga Pradipika. Munger, India: Bihar School of Yoga, 1985, pg. 177 (Chapter II, 5).

[116] Desikachar, TKV. Yogayajnavalkya Samhita. Chennai: Krishnamacharya Yoga Mandiram, 2000, pg. 43.

[117] Krishnamacharya, Yogacarya T. Sri Nathamuni's Yogarahasya. Chennai: Krishnamacharya Yoga Mandiram, 1998, pg. 52.

[118] Swami Kuvalayananda and Swami Digambarji. Vasistha Samhita. Lonavla, India: Kaivalyadhama, 1969, pg. 14.

[119] Swami Muktibodhananda Saraswati. Hatha Yoga Pradipika. Bihar School of Yoga, Munger, India, 1985, pg. 272.

[120] Mala SrivatsanSrivatsa quoting T. Krishnamacharya in "Guru Parampara". Darsanam magazine, Madras: Krishnamacharya Yoga Mandiram, Nov. 1995 (Vol. 4 No. 3), pg. 39.

[121] Mukunda Stiles. Yoga Sutras of Patanjali. Boston: Weiser, 2001, pg. 9.

[122] TKV Desikachar. Health, Healing & Beyond. NY: Aperture, 1998, pg. 169-170.

[123] Swami Venkatesananda. The Supreme Yoga - Yoga Vasistha. Chiltern Yoga Trust: South Freemantle, Western Australia, 1984, pg. 295.

[124] Avraham Greenbaum. The Wings of the Sun. Traditional Jewish Healing in Theory and Practice. Jerusalem: Breslov Research Institute, 1995, back cover.

[125] Talks with Sri Ramana Maharshi, Tiruvannamalai, India: T.N. Venkataraman, 1994, pg. 583.

[126] The Spiritual Teachings of Ramana Maharshi. Boston: Shambhala, 1988, pg. 3.

[127] Swami Venkatesananda. The Supreme Yoga - Yoga Vasistha. Chiltern Yoga Trust: South Freemantle, Western Australia, 1984, pg. 295.

[128] Geeta Iyengar. "Yoga and Ayurveda". Yoga '87. San Francisco: Iyengar Yoga Conference magazine, pg. 45.

[129] TKV Desikachar. "Krishnamacharya: The Yogi and Teacher". Darsanam magazine, Madras: Krishnamacharya Yoga Mandiram, Aug. 1992 (Vol. 1 No. 2), pg. 14.

[130] Jaideva Singh. Siva Sutras. Delhi: Motilal Banarsidass, 1979.

[131] Twelve Steps and Twelve Traditions. NY: Alcoholics Anonymous World Services, Inc., 1981, pg. 41.

[132] Candace Pert. Molecules of Emotion. pg. 265.

[133] Swami Nityaswarupananda. Astavakra Samhita (II, 8). Calcutta: Advaita Ashrama, 1975, pg. 21.

[134] T.K.V. Desikachar. The Heart of Yoga. Rochester, VT: Inner Traditions International, 1995, pg. 54.

[135] Mukunda Stiles. <u>Yoga Sutras of Patanjali</u>. Boston: Weiser Books, 2002, pg. 3.

[136] Indra Devi. <u>Yoga for You</u>. Salt Lake City: Gibbs Smith Publisher, 2002, pg. 44.

[137] Harish Johari. <u>Breath, Mind, and Consciousness</u>. Rochester, VT: Destiny Books, 1989, pg. 3.

[138] Wynn Kapit, Robert Macey, Esmail Meisami. <u>The Physiology Coloring Book</u>. NY: Harper Collins Publishers, 1987, pg. 105.

[139] In my many talks with physicians and a survey of physiology texts, this reflex is not mentioned. I would be most interested to learn of an explanation of this reflex.

[140] James Funderburk. <u>Science Studies Yoga</u>. Honesdale, PA: Himalayan International Institute of Yoga Science and Philosophy, 1977, pg. 49.

[141] Swami Muktibodhananda Saraswati. <u>Swara Yoga</u>. Bihar: Bihar School of Yoga , 1984, pg. 138-139.

[142] Harish Johari. <u>Breath, Mind, and Consciousness</u>. Rochester, VT: Destiny Books, 1989, pg. 54 quoting from Brain Mind Bulletin, Vol. 8, No. 3, Jan. 3, 1983.

[143] <u>Ibid</u>, pg. 2.

[144] Blanche Phillips Howard. <u>Dance of the Self - Movements for Body, Mind and Spirit</u>. New York: Simon and Schuster, 1974, pg. 21-22.

[145] David Frawley. Mukunda Stiles, editor. <u>New England Institute of Ayurvedic Medicine</u>. Manual #2. Boston: NEIAM, 1999, pg. 1.

[146] Mukunda Stiles. <u>Yoga Sutras of Patanjali</u>. Boston: Weiser Books, 2002, pg. 11.

[147] Swami Venkatesananda. <u>Vasistha's Yoga</u>. NY: SUNY Press, 1993, pg. 641.

[148] <u>Ibid.</u> pg. 2.

[149] Ram Karan Sharma and Vaidya Bhagwan Dash. <u>Agnivesa's Caraka Samhita</u>. Varanasi: Chowkhamba Sanskrit Series Office, 1976, pg. 25.

[150] There are no Ayurvedic medical schools outside of India. Many Ayurvedic practitioners are being training in the West but there are no Ayurvedic physicians except those who have graduated from Ayurvedic medical colleges in India. To this date only one westerner, Robert Svoboda, is a fully qualified Ayurvedic physician.

[151] R. Prabhakar. "Nathamuni's Yoga" in The Yoga Review, vol. I, no. 3, 1981, pg. 135.

XIV. Recommended Readings

Copeland, Paul. Beginning Yoga. Published by the author, Davis, Ca., 1973. Vinyasa sequences given the author from private studies with Krishnamacharya in 1971-72.

_____. A Continuation of the Teachings of T. Krishnamacharya. Published by the author, Davis, Ca ., l974. Intermediate Vinyasas and a summary of pranayamas with bandhas.

Cousens, Gabriel, M.D. Spiritual Nutrition and the Rainbow Diet. A scientific and spiritual autobiographical account of how multi-dimension bodies receive nourishment.

Desikachar, Kausthub. The Yoga of the Yogi. Chennai: Krishnamacharya Yoga Mandiram, 2005.

Insights into adapting to individuals by the masters grandson.

Desikachar, T.K.V. with R.H. Cravens. Health, Healing and Beyond. Aperture, Denville, NJ, 1998. A

detailed biography of Krishnamacharya and his teaching methods.

Douillard, John. The 3-Season Diet. New York: Harmony Books, 2000. A helpful diet for applying Ayurvedic principles to the changes of the seasons for maintaining energy balance.

_____. Dr. John Douillard's Ayurvedic Pulse Reading Course. Boulder, CO: Lifespa, 1998.

Frawley, David. Ayurveda and the Mind. The Healing of Consciousness. Lotus Press, Twin Lakes, Perspectives on what is the mind, consciousness and Yoga psychotherapy.

_____. Yoga and Ayurveda – Self-Healing and Self-Realization. Lotus Press, Twin Lakes, An excellent perspective on the interrelationship for an integrated lifestyle.

Johari, Harish. Dhanwantari – A Complete Guide to the Ayurvedic Life. Rochester, VT: Healing Arts Press, 1998. A Tantrik masters point of view.

Lad, Vasant. Ayurveda - The Science of Self-Healing. Lotus Press, Wilmot, WI, 1984. Graphically portrays individual needs for optimal health.

Ranade, Subash & Sunanda. Ayurveda and Yoga Therapy. Pune: Anmol Prakashan, 1995. A good beginning although a "cook book" approach to integrating these approaches to treating diseases.

Sharma, Ram Karan Dr. and Vaidya Bhagwan Dash. Agnivesa's Caraka Samhita. 4 volumes. Chowkhamba Sanskrit Series Office, Varanasi, India, 1976. The original text of Ayurveda translated into English covers all aspects of health.

Stiles, Mukunda. With Great Respect and Love - Yoga Sutras of Patanjali. Boston: Weiser Books, 2002. A devotional rendition free of commentary.

Svoboda, Robert E., Dr. Prakruti - Your Ayurvedic Constitution. Geocom Limited, Albuquerque, New Mexico, l988. I recommended this or his other as a first book on Ayurveda.

Ayurveda for Women. Rochester, VT: Healing Arts Press, 2000. Help for women of all ages with herbal and food guidelines.

Swami Muktananda. Meditate. Albany: State University of New York Press, 1980. A powerful voice on the innate drive for spirituality and an excellent guide for all meditators.

Swami Venkatesananda. Vasistha's Yoga. Albany, NY: SUNY Press, 1993. A treasure house of   spiritual wisdom, according to Swami Muktananda, leading step by step to illumination.

Tiwari, Bri. Maya. The Path of Practice. NY: Ballantine Books, 2000. Women's spiritual practices for healing, the breath of life, sound as medicine, and feeding the soul.

Verma, Vinod. Patanjali and Ayurvedic Yoga. Delhi: Motilal Banarsidass, 2001. More theoretical than practical by an Indian scientist.

XX. Appendix Charts

Ayurvedic Charts

	Vata	Pitta	Kapha
Elements	Air and ether	Fire and water	Earth and water
Sense	Touch, hearing	Sight	Smell, taste
Spiritual Guide	Sarasvati, Brahma	Kali, Shiva	Lakshmi, Vishnu
Subtle Energy	Prana	Tejas	Ojas
Qualities	Dry, cool, light irregular, mobile, permeating	Slightly oily, hot, light, intense, fluid, penetrating	Oily, cold, heavy, stable, firm
Region	Pelvic cavity	Abdominal region	Head, neck
Polluted site	Bones, thighs, legs,	Blood, sweat, lymph	Joints, stomach, fat
Home	Large intestine	Small intestine	Heart
Time of day	2-6 am & pm Dawn and dusk	10am-2pm & 10pm-2am Sun above & below	6-10 am & pm Sun mid-range
Purpose	Start things	Organize things	Finish
Function	Motion, rhythm	Assimilation	Structure, strength

Factors creating imbalance

	Vata	Pitta	Kapha
Root of Disease	Desire, lust	Pride, hatred	Closed mindedness
Detrimental Factors	Too much exercise, fasting, late hours, travel, rain	Over work, sunbathe, irregular eating, alcohol, summer	Sleeping in day, over eating, cold foods, winter
Signs of Imbalance	Throbbing, shooting, migrating	Burning, pulling, sucking	Dull ache, mild, heaviness
Common Diseases	Osteoarthritis, cold extremities, motion sickness, hypertension, hypoglycemia, constipation	Inflammatory arthritis, acne, repeated fevers, hepatitis, ulcer	Edema, diabetes, kidney stones, asthma, heart conditions, constipation

Signs of Imbalance

Vata	Pitta	Kapha
Fear	Anger	Attachment
Anxiety	Frustration	Opinions
Stress	Impatience	Self-centered

Signs of clarity

Vata	Pitta	Kapha
Rote learning – repetition	Seeing clearly	Grasping
Understanding	Knowing	Opinionated
Intuitive	Discernment	Devoted to learning

AYURVEDIC YOGA THERAPY

Purpose: To experience the Divine Self as your own self
by balancing doshas to draw your mind to its root.

		Vata	Pitta	Kapha
Treatment		relaxation	discrimination	detoxification
		rhythmic exercise	enthusiasm	strength promoting
		self knowledge	self discipline	devotion, love
Attitude		seek balance	zest, joy	devotion
Ideal Tastes (in order)		salty, sour,	bitter, sweet,	pungent, bitter,
		sweet	astringent	astringent
Main meal		dinner before sunset	lunch	breakfast
Diet		cooked vegetables	vegetables, fruit,	vegetables best food,
		lt. poultry/fish-	grains, ideal to be a vegetarian	limit quantity of food
		likely to need animal protein		
Beneficial Actions		massage, sunbathe, silent meditation, drink warm water	volunteer, teamwork, give blood, hugs, water play, walking at night, moon bathe	vigorous exercise, devotional singing, walking, swimming, sunbathe

Method of exercise	slow, silent rhythmic motion with breath	moderate-intense invigorating	challenging, holding to increase strength
Yoga Sadhana	raja, Jnana	tantra, karma	hatha, Bhakti
Yoga practice	*Joint Freeing Series,	solar series,	*Shoulderstand,
	balancing poses,	*gentle, long twists	bridge, lion pose,
	knee to chest,	boat, bow,	fish, peacock,
	*Yoga Nidra,	sphinx pose,	Warrior Vinyasa,
	*Palm tree Vinyasa	Sunbird Vinyasa	*Sun salute long
	Sun salute slow	*Sun salute moderate	
Pranayama	*ujjaye breathing	*Bhastrika	*Kapalabhati
Mudra	Jnana	Tara	Anjali
Mantra	So'ham	ma vidvisavahai	IstadeVata (chosen deity)
Perfections	zest for life,	desire for change,	extroversion,
	contentment,	discrimination,	wisdom, assertive,
	patience, courage	introspection,	determined effort,
		enthusiasm	laughter, joy

*best

Ayurvedic Yoga Therapy Course Outline

Sequence of Events within a Class

For Teachers – WELCOME EVERYONE PERSONALLY
Mentally offer the fruits to God – whatever happens is Her doing
Centering on your Self with deep breathing into wave breath

Introductory Mantras and/or Invocation to Yoga
Self-Observation (svadhyaya) – what's up today, what do you need?
Invocation - "With great respect and love I honor my Heart, my inner teacher
- Namaskar"
Readings from the Yoga Sutras
Preparatory exercises - Joint Freeing Series -Pavanmuktasana
Strength Isolation Exercises
Vinyasa Sequences – flowing poses
Structural Yoga Poses – Static Asanas
Restorative Poses and Yoga Nidra - Deep Relaxation - Savasana
Energetic Breathing and Healing – Pranayama
Purification – Kriyas (tapas) – cleansing the body and senses
Pratyahara – Mudras – training of the senses
Meditation and Devotional Practices (Isvara-pranidhana)
Closing Mantras and/or Universal Prayer
For Teachers – "THANK YOU - for allowing me to serve you"

About the Author

Mukunda Stiles, one of the American pioneers in Yoga Therapy, created his Structural Yoga Therapy system in 1976 following his training in Krishnamacharya's lineage of teachers; most notably Rama Jyoti Vernon, BKS Iyengar and Indra Devi. He has a BA in religious studies with a thesis on the Yoga Sutras and did graduate study in kinesiology and therapeutic exercise. From 1974 until 1982 he served on the staff of four ashrams under the guidance of Swami Muktananda. He is the author of the best seller Structural Yoga Therapy, the Yoga Sutras of Patanjali and has edited 7 books on Ayurveda. His rendition of the Yoga Sutras was praised by Iyengar, Baba Hari Dass, and David Frawley. Mukunda is a contributing author to the anthology The Marriage of Sex and Spirit. He is currently working on a fourth book Classical Yoga Meditation - Practices from the Yoga Sutras. Mukunda trains spiritual mentors with the Claritas Institute, directed by Joan Borysenko. NEW – His spiritual mentoring process is featured in her book Your Soul's Compass – What is Spiritual Guidance? He is on the Board of Advisors for the International Association of Yoga Therapists. His website www.yogatherapycenter.org describes his offerings at his home in Holyoke, Massachusetts and at training sites throughout the US and Europe.

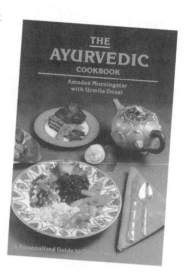

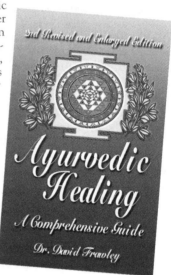

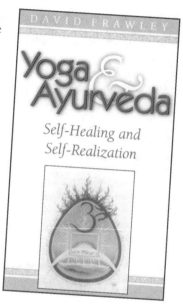

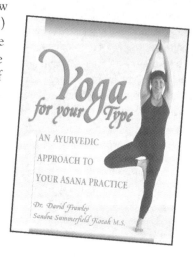

Ayurvedic Cooking
for Westerners

by Amadea Morningstar

Ayurvedic Cooking for Westerners offers familiar Western foods lovingly prepared with Ayurvedic principles. Learn how to cook fresh, easy to make recipes for healthy folks, as well as those with illnesses, including allergies and candida. Written by Amadea Morningstar, co-author of the best-selling, *The Ayurvedic Cookbook*, this book is certain to open wide the door to this ancient East Indian, yet universal system of healing and nourishment, with more than 230 new and delicious Ayurvedic recipes.

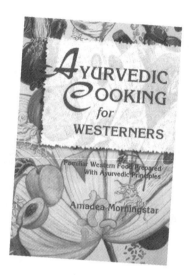

Trade Paper   ISBN 978-0-9149-5514-6   395 pp $19.95

Available at bookstores and natural food stores nationwide or order your copy directly by sending $19.95 plus $2.50 shipping/handling ($1.50 s/h for each additional copy ordered at the same time) to:

Lotus Press, P O Box 325, Twin Lakes, WI 53181 USA
toll free order line: 800 824 6396 office phone: 262 889 8561
office fax: 262 889 8591 email: lotuspress@lotuspress.com
web site: www.lotuspress.com

Lotus Press is the publisher of a wide range of books and software in the field of alternative health, including Ayurveda, Chinese medicine, herbology, aromatherapy, Reiki and energetic healing modalities. Request our free book catalog.

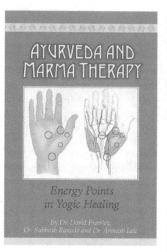